Judith Wills is one of the country's most popular diet and fitness writers. As well as being the author of the bestselling *A Flat Stomach in Fifteen Days* (Sphere, 1990) she also has a weekly slimming column in the *Daily Express* and is a regular broadcaster on TV and radio.

High Speed Slimming

The Revolutionary Diet for Fast, Safe and Permanent Weight Loss

JUDITH WILLS

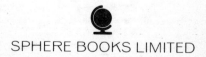

SPHERE BOOKS LIMITED

A Sphere Book

First published in Great Britain by Sphere Books Ltd
1992
Reprinted 1992

A CIP catalogue record for this book
is available from the British Library

ISBN 0 7474 1016 X

Typeset by Leaper & Gard Ltd, Bristol, England
Printed and bound in Great Britain by
Cox & Wyman Ltd, Reading

Sphere Books Ltd
A Division of
Macdonald & Co (Publishers) Ltd
165 Great Dover Street
London SE1 4YA

Contents

Introduction

Last year, over a third of readers taking part in an annual survey for one slimming magazine said that their main reason for giving up on a diet was *not* the sight of a chocolate bar, *not* the aroma of home-baked pie, *not* the promise of a free meal at a Michelin-starred restaurant – but the fact that they weren't losing weight quickly enough. One large slimming club organization which gave its members a questionnaire asking what makes the perfect diet discovered that most members valued quick weight loss above almost any other aspect of dieting.

I'm not surprised. If there's one thing almost as bad as being overweight, it's starting a low-calorie diet, sometimes an extremely low-calorie diet, and suffering misery – as many diets will make you do – but sticking to it, only to find that the scales show a disappointingly low weight loss. The pain hardly seems worth it. Then a helpful member of the family accuses you of cheating and sooner or later – usually sooner – you give up the wretched diet.

Research shows that people who record a good, fast weight loss are much, much more likely to stick to a diet right down to their target weight. I also know that people promised a fast weight loss are more likely to start that diet in the first place. Such a diet has to be good news for the several million of us in this country who are overweight.

So why is it, then, that rapid weight loss is often looked upon by some doctors, nutritionists and many slimming experts as undesirable? In the '60s and '70s, 'fad' and 'crash' diets were all the rage. But by the '80s more and more experts were beginning to say that rapid weight loss might not be a good idea. It could be dangerous, said the pundits, and very often after 'crash' dieting, the weight would return almost as quickly as it had disappeared.

Believe it or not, as one of the country's top diet experts I have said that kind of thing myself, many, many times, in the past. So, over the last few years, most responsible dieting advice has been to lose weight slowly, with 1-2 lbs/450-900 g a week most frequently mentioned as the ideal amount to lose.

However, two facts have recently made me take a new look at the whole business of quick weight loss. Firstly, I appreciate people's obvious wish to lose weight faster than that 1-2 lbs/450-900 g a week. Many people simply choose to stay fat rather than stick to a slow and tedious diet — and all those people who DO choose to stay fat are putting their health at risk and possibly shortening their lives. Obesity is a real health hazard. If you're 20% or more over your right weight — that is, for instance, if you weigh

12 stone/76 kg when you should weigh 10 stone/ 63.5 kg — you are increasing your risk of heart disease, circulatory problems and high blood pressure, diabetes, arthritis in the weight-bearing joints and a variety of other problems. And the longer you continue to be overweight — or the more weight you put on — the greater the risk you are running. Secondly, I realized that most of the professional objections to losing weight fast were really objections to the *means* by which most people were doing it – that is, on very low-calorie and often nutritionally unsound diets; diets which I, too, would be the first to condemn.

So I set about finding out, first of all, just what was so terrible about losing weight faster than a pound or two a week and, secondly, whether it would be practical or feasible to shed the pounds fast without risking health, life or sanity. I am now sure that I have discovered the answer — no, there is nothing terrible about fast weight loss done the right way. And yes, there is a way you can do it sensibly.

The results of my research are here in this book. Let me first repeat myself by saying: I do not believe in, or ask you to follow, mad 'crash' diets. I do not believe it necessary to go lower than 800 calories a day on any slimming diet. I do not expect or want you to follow a boring, liquids-only diet, or to take pills or potions, or even vitamin supplements of any kind, to speed weight loss. You can achieve high speed weight loss without the need to worry about what it is doing to your body or health.

High Speed Slimming will help you to lose up to half a stone in a week – many people will be able to shed a stone in as little as 14 days. I can virtually guarantee that anyone can lose at least 3-4 lbs / 1.5-2.0 kg a week every week if the methods I describe in this book are followed completely – without an extremely low-calorie diet, without any risk to your health and, probably most important of all, without putting it all back on again quickly as soon as the diet is over.

Everything you need to know for *safe* and *speedy* weight loss – and a permanently slim future – is here in this book. So what are you waiting for?

CHAPTER ONE

Rapid Weight Loss – A Fat Lot of Good?

'The worst thing you can do is diet too fast.'

'Lose weight quickly and it will come back quickly.'

'Crash dieting will make you ill.'

'You should never lose weight at more than 1-2 lbs a week.'

I found these remarks – and plenty more similar to them – in just a quick glance through some women's magazines and some free health education leaflets one day last year. There is no doubt that over the past decade, rapid weight loss, crash and fad diets have all had a tough time – in the media, on TV, and via doctors, health educators and nutritionists. Although I intend to show you how you can achieve speedy weight loss without any hint of a crash diet or a fad diet, rapid loss has come to be firmly associated in our minds with very low-calorie senseless dieting. It's taken for granted that if anyone is losing weight quickly, he or she must be following some mad, bad regime.

Why? Well, let's look back at the history of diets

and dieting over the past thirty years or so to answer that question. After the literally lean times of the war years, the '50s were the celebratory years when people gladly ate all that they could, grateful to have choice and plenty once again. Dieting was the last thing on our minds. In the early '60s, however, suddenly it became fashionable to be thin like top models Twiggy and The Shrimp. Legs in the new mini-skirts had to be long and skinny and cheekbones had to show, otherwise you were not 'in'.

A similar thing was happening in the States, where diet books began reaching the bestseller lists with ease and outselling almost everything else. *The Mayo Clinic Diet* was one of the first and – like many that were to follow, such as the million-selling *Scarsdale Diet* – was based on a way of eating that is now considered nutritionally unsound, the low-carbohydrate principle.

WHEN BREAD WAS BANNED ...

The high-protein diets fashionable in the '60s (such as *Dr Atkins Diet Revolution*) were high in protein – and cholesterol-rich foods, such as eggs and meat – and very low in the carbohydrates now known to be such an important part of a healthy diet, such as bread, potatoes and rice, and some were also high in FAT. The classic diet meal of the '60s was a grilled steak with a pat of butter and a green side salad.

Bread and potatoes were nothing more than distant memories for the typical dieter of the day.

These low-carbohydrate diets were popular because they did often achieve high initial weight losses. What people didn't realize was that much of this initial loss was fluid – a side-effect of such a drastic reduction in carbohydrate which normally literally acts like a sponge in the body to soak up fluid weighing several pounds. Such popular American diets formed the basis of a thousand fad and crash diets in the UK in the '60s and '70s. Looking back through my files and bookshelves, I find plenty of examples – let's look at a few of the more bizarre ones.

Firstly, we have a day's eating from a 'Five-Day Mixed Diet' in a book called *Successful Slimming* published in the '70s. The diet allows around 850 calories for this day with the only carbohydrate coming in the form of alcohol (not the right sort of carbohydrate!) and a very tiny amount of green vegetables. In other words, almost all the calories in the diet are protein and fat. The introduction says that the sherry is allowed as a 'bit of an uplift' (it would probably have the reverse effect) and the only other drink allowed, including water, is two cups of lemon tea.

Breakfast: 1 boiled egg and 1 natural yogurt.
11 o'clock: 2oz/56g Dutch cheese, 1 glass dry sherry.
2 o'clock: 4oz/113g steak, raw or grilled, lettuce salad, lemon tea.

5 o'clock: 2oz/56g Dutch cheese, 1 glass dry sherry.

8 o'clock: plate of boiled greens, lemon tea.

Apart from being decidedly unpalatable, this diet has a carbohydrate-protein-fat ratio of 18%-54%-28% – almost the complete opposite of today's diet recommendations, which are a carbohydrate level of 50-60% (of total calories), a protein level of 15% and a fat level of 25-35%. Recent research indicates that the higher the carbohydrate and the lower the fat in the diet, the easier it is to lose weight, which is why my own *High Speed Slimming* diet goes one better and has a ratio of 60-20-20. But more of that later! Back to those crazy early diets.

In the same book, *Successful Slimming*, there is a diet to help you lose a stone in 10 days which allows you approximately 600 calories a day from milk, meat, egg, a very little chicken or fish, salad and greens, fruit juice and coffee – and that's it.

As these basic low-carbohydrate diets eventually got boring through repetition, so the diet ideas produced got more and more faddy to try to keep the public's interest. One popular columnist of the day writing for a national newspaper devised a diet of approximately 700 calories to lose 2½lbs/1.1kg in one day, consisting of six glasses of champagne, four whole grapefruits and one cup of black coffee! I can hardly imagine the upset stomachs, dehydration headaches and empty purses which must have been caused by that one! The same writer also relayed the world's cheapest diet from Scandinavia – you drank up to two pints of water a day in which 2 lbs/900 g of unpeeled potatoes had been boiled.

THE YO-YO

By this time, millions of people in the Western world – especially women – were hooked on the idea of dieting, but discovering that, sadly, these fad diet regimes were not actually helping many people to slim down in the long term. A new phrase, 'the yo-yo dieter', was coined for all the thousands of people who lost weight but soon gave up, or lost weight and put it straight back on again. Then they would begin a new crash diet and repeat the pattern, often over and over and over again. It's a pattern that even today has stuck with many of those early dieters, women and some men now in their middle age and permanently on the dieting see-saw.

At least the more iron-willed dieters got down to their target weight. Many others never did – one diet after another would be abandoned with the would-be slimmer complaining of hunger, dizziness, tiredness, bad temper and deprivation. 'Oh, I haven't got the willpower to stick to a diet,' would come the cry. Yet it wasn't people's willpower at fault, but rather the types of diet on offer that were to blame.

THE LOW BLOOD SUGAR SYNDROME

As we've seen, most of these diets were woefully short of both carbohydrate and calories and any diet which falls too short of either of these will be a diet that induces failure. Such diets are hard to stick to for a simple physical reason – they produce a physical side-effect called hypoglycaemia, commonly known as low blood sugar.

The body fluid, the loss of which is associated with a low-carbohydrate diet as I explained above, contains a substance called glycogen – a form of glucose. Glycogen is what the body uses as 'instant' energy. If the body's glycogen store is depleted by a low-carbohydrate diet and if the body is not receiving any glucose via the diet, the result is low blood sugar and very real accompanying symptoms – headache, tiredness, weakness, lack of vitality and, quite often, a physical craving for a high-carbohydrate food. This is not weak willpower on the part of the dieter but simply the body crying out for what it needs. And it is why the dieter will break the diet with a chocolate bar or cake rather than with a ham sandwich – the sugary chocolate bar or cake will provide instant energy because it will be converted very quickly into blood glucose. Because the average dieter doesn't understand this physical need, he or she feels guilty and gives up dieting in despair.

WE *DID* BELIEVE IN MIRACLES

By the late '70s all those failed dieters and dis-appointing diets had done little to dull the national craving for yet more silly diets, and by now the diet peddlers had really put on their thinking caps. To keep people interested, they invented 'miracle food' diets.

Hence we had the grapefruit diet (eat half a grapefruit before every meal and it will 'burn up' the calories in your meal, we were told). We had the Beverly Hills pineapple diet (the miracle enzymes in pineapples would also burn off our calories in a very special way, we were told). Then there was the revival of *The Hay System* (never mix protein foods and carbohydrate foods at the same meal, we were told, because the one interferes with the proper digestion of the other). Then there were the miracle tea diets, miracle starch-blocker pill diets and, of course, the advent of the very low-calorie liquid protein diets which, in their original formula back in the '70s, allegedly caused several deaths in the USA.

Weren't we a gullible lot? Needless to say, all of these diets were just as hard to stick to as the earlier crash diets and many were as dubious nutritionally. No wonder, then, that we reached the start of the '80s with crash diets and fast weight loss having a bad name – diets which had done nothing but kept us, as a nation, just as fat as we were before.

THE ANTI-DIET YEARS

So came the 'anti-diet' backlash. Nutritionists, doctors, slimming clubs, it seemed everyone began bad-mouthing the 'get slim quick' idea and promoting the idea that instead the only way to lose weight was to do it slowly on a healthy, well-balanced diet. First in January 1983 came a report on obesity from the Royal College of Physicians which said that 'the public needs to recognize that crash diets are in the short term dangerous and do little to help them adjust permanently ... to maintain weight loss'. Then came the COMA (Committee on Medical Aspects of Food Policy) Report later in 1983 which stressed the importance of eating a healthy, reduced-fat diet including plenty of unrefined carbohydrates. Finally the book *Dieting Makes You Fat* was published, also in 1983, telling us all that repeated low-calorie dieting was a fool's game. It claimed that low-calorie diets caused us to lose too much lean body tissue – i.e. muscle – and that continual diets would slow down our metabolic rate and make it even harder to lose weight next time. This, it seemed, set the seal on the fate of all crash diets known to man.

From 1984 onwards, slow but sure, very sensible 'non-diet-diets' have been in vogue. For a while, indeed, the very word 'diet' became a four-letter word and any would-be slimmer was hard pushed to find a diet anywhere that would lose him or her weight at a rate faster than 2 lbs/900 g a week.

The only diet book to make a big impression in the '80s was *The F-Plan* which – you guessed it – advocated steady weight loss on a diet high in sensible fibre and low in fat.

I have to say now that throughout the '80s I was editor of one of the country's top slimming magazines and I was just as enthusiastic in condemning crash diets as anyone else was.

THE LIQUID LUNCH CRAZE

And yet despite all this bad publicity, there was still a big market for whatever very low-calorie diets were still around. Fast weight loss was still, despite everything, what people really wanted. This was why the phenomenally successful *Cambridge Diet* took off in the UK in the '80s. Three milk shakes a day, all the nutrients you needed and massive weight loss – these were the promises and people literally lapped the product up.

Why? Simple. Although the nutritional content of most of the new, 'slow and steady' diets was undoubtedly a huge improvement on all the '60s diets, these new sensible 'plans' weren't working any better to get us slim than the old crash diets had! We were still, by 1990, just as fat as a nation, according to government statistics, as we had been in 1980!

Though 'slow and steady' is a lovely idea, such regimes often fail, I am sure, not because they induce problems such as low blood sugar or hunger pangs — but because they take no account of human nature. Who wants to carry on dieting when the scales show such a small loss that you can hardly see it? No-one does. It is only quick results — and a good continuing weight loss — that keep people keen to diet and keep them motivated. The Weight Watchers organization began its *Quick Success* programme a few years ago after it surveyed its members and discovered that fast results were what they wanted above everything else.

The very low-calorie liquid diets — such as the *Cambridge Diet* — went from strength to strength in the '80s (having been re-formulated since those early days when they were blamed for deaths in the USA) and they are still popular today. I confess that I am not a great liquid diet fan other than for very short-term use or to replace one meal a day rather than two or three. So many dieters have told me how mind-numbingly boring they find these diets day in, day out — and there is no need to go anywhere near as low as 400 or so calories a day to achieve fabulous weight losses. I also dislike the idea of grossly obese people — with many stones to lose — being fed a diet of only 400 or 500 calories a day without the supervision of a doctor — it is a scientific fact that the fatter you are, the more you can eat and still lose weight.

And yet the government said, in its 1987 report on these very low-calorie liquid diets (VLCDs) that they don't recommend people with a body mass index of 25 or less (people with only a little weight to lose) should use VLCDs. (Body mass index is another way of judging obesity rather than using height/weight charts, and a person of average weight has a BMI of 20–25.) The same report also recommended that no one should use a VLCD for more than 3 or 4 weeks at a time as the sole source of nutrition – with the implication that people in the middle-range of over-weight, say with a couple of stones to lose, should also not use a VLCD from start to finish of their diet.

VLCDs, then, obviously have only limited use for most would-be dieters. I don't doubt they have their place, though, and their popularity has simply rein-forced the fact that most of us have reached the stage where we would rather stay fat than read one more diet feature telling us to lose it slowly. And yet that is exactly what we are continually being told. The message we are still receiving is re-educate yourself to healthier eating habits, less fat, more fibre, slow weight loss …'

So, what is the average overweight person to do who wants to lose weight now and lose it quickly, but who doesn't want to run the risk of ill health, and definitely doesn't want to diet only to put the weight all back on again? Is there an answer?

Yes, there is. I can guarantee – to all the people who have been yo-yo dieters; to all the people who have begun diets that have never gone beyond Day 2; to all the people who have tried the 'slow and sure' way and got disillusioned at minimal results; to everyone who is overweight and has not even tried to diet after seeing how much pain and misery their dieting friends go through to achieve so little; and to all the people who claim they can't lose weight on 1000 calories a day – to you all, I say that you can lose weight faster than that 1-2 lbs/450-900g a week without any need to worry and without resorting to any of the fad and bad methods I've described earlier in this chapter.

Because, you see, what most of the critics (including myself) of fast weight loss have really been criticizing all these years is not the rapidity of the loss itself, but the methods used to achieve that loss, i.e. strictly limiting calories to less than 800 a day – even sometimes down to virtually no calories a day – and at the same time strictly limiting the possibility of getting all the nutrients people need for good health and well-being.

All that deprivation and risk to health, followed by what seems like inevitable and equally rapid putting back on of the weight lost – on the face of it, it does all seem like a silly, pointless exercise, doesn't it? But if we can find a way of changing the methods by which you lose weight quickly, there will be no dieters – or experts – left to complain.

As I am about to show you in the next chapter, I believe that the critics of fast weight loss have totally missed this vital distinction. I will also explain how new research has disproved the 'dieting makes you fat' theory – fast weight loss does not slow down your metabolic rate long term any more than slow weight loss does and neither does it predispose the dieter to put weight back on quickly or to lose more than normal amounts of lean body tissue.

My *High Speed Slimming* method involves not only a diet that manages to be both sensible and, in its own way, quite revolutionary, but also some important lifestyle modifications to help speed up the rate at which you burn calories, along with an entertaining exercise routine which uses all the latest research to maximize your fat-burning potential.

Diet, lifestyle and exercise: these are the three keys to a quickly slim – and permanently slim – you.

CHAPTER TWO

Fast and Safe

So you want to lose weight – and lose it quickly. Don't feel guilty about that. Once you have made the decision that you need to lose weight and really want to slim yourself down, it makes nothing but sense to make a positive effort that will bring positive results.

So let's sum up the major reasons why you will benefit from losing weight quickly.

BENEFITS OF RAPID WEIGHT LOSS

A fast start gives encouragement

From talking to hundreds of successful slimmers, I know that it was seeing their fat disappear fast in the early weeks that gave them the incentive to continue. Finding their 'fat' clothes hanging loose after a week or so, seeing inches shrink away from hips and waist, having people compliment them on their weight loss.

Immediate results are what get dieters started. A pound or two a week just doesn't show – especially if you have a lot of weight to lose.

Continuing quick weight loss gives incentive to carry on

After asking dozens of failed dieters why they had given up trying to lose weight, I discovered that the most common reason was, 'It was bad enough sticking to the diet – but the weight came off so slowly, it hardly seemed worth the effort.'

Many, many slimmers can get halfway to their target weight without much trouble – but they never manage to lose the last bit. Fast weight loss diets get more people down to target than do slow weight loss diets.

You will soon be a 'normal' person

If you lose your excess weight quickly, it stands to reason that the day will come sooner when you can get on with your life as an ordinary, non-dieting person. You can stop worrying about being fat or thin, and start enjoying life … looking good and feeling good. Being fat tends to take over lives – the fat person can think of nothing but being slim 'one day'. Once you are slim, there is so much more time for enjoying yourself.

So isn't it great that I can tell you now that there is no need to feel ashamed in any way that you want to slim fast, and there is no need to feel that you will be doing your body any harm at all by losing weight quickly?

In the last chapter we heard all about why fast weight loss has got such a bad name over the past years. Now let's take the criticisms one by one and see just how the *High Speed Slimming* method avoids all of them.

I don't want you to skip this bit – I want you, the potential high-speed slimmer, to read it all thoroughly because I want you to trust *High Speed Slimming*; I want you to feel secure and happy with my methods and look forward to beginning what I am sure will be the last diet of your life.

Let's look at the criticisms in turn.

STANDARD CRITICISMS

'Fast weight loss could be dangerous to my health.'

Very low-calorie diets can be dangerous for two reasons. Firstly, any very drastic reduction in calorie consumption – especially in very big, heavy people – can put great stress on the body and its organs, particularly the heart. So for the thousands of over-weight people who already suffer from illnesses such as high blood pressure and heart and circulatory problems, following a very low-calorie unbalanced diet could lead to trouble. And more minor problems, such as dizziness, faintness, tiredness and lack of concentration are frequently reported side effects of diets that are too low in calories.

However, *High Speed Slimming* does not involve any drastic reduction in the number of calories you consume. It slims you quickly by using the opposite approach — by increasing your metabolic rate. Also, your calorie consumption is tailored to your own needs — the more overweight you are, the more you eat. And, because I know that reducing calories more than necessary is just a waste of time, you will never be down to near-fasting levels. The lowest anyone goes is 800 calories a day — some people will diet on as much as 1,500 calories a day. And I am sure that you will feel fitter and healthier on this diet and exercise plan than on anything you have tried before.

The second reason very low-calorie diets may be dangerous is that they may cause ill health by not providing you with all the nutrients that your body needs. We all need a certain amount of carbohydrate, protein, a little fat, and all the essential vitamins and minerals, as well as water, to survive in a healthy state.

If you follow a nutritionally unbalanced diet for a day or two you are unlikely to come to any great harm. But follow one for weeks on end, and you almost certainly will. Sadly all too many diets, even today, are not balanced and do not contain all you need for good health. Many are short on complex carbohydrates — the grains, root vegetables, pulses, fresh fruit and vegetables — that we all need for health. Shortage of these can lead to digestive problems, constipation and perhaps even bowel disease and there is also evidence linking low carbohydrate diets with cancer and heart disease.

A diet that is too low in protein may affect your vital organs and your body's ability to renew its lean tissue – especially if such a diet is combined with a lot of exercise.

A diet that cuts out all fat can also cause problems. We don't need lots of fat, especially animal fat, but we do still need a certain amount of the three groups of fat – saturated, monosaturated and poly-unsaturated. Many of the very low-fat diets around may not be as healthy as they seem. Mono- and poly-unsaturated fats lower blood cholesterol, while a small amount of saturated fat keeps the body in balance.

Furthermore, many slimming diets are very low in calcium-rich foods, such as dairy produce. Calcium is essential to maintain bone. Many diets also cut down on foods rich in B vitamins, such as lean red meats. I've analysed dozens of diets on offer in magazines and books and found most of them short of at least some vital nutrients.

In the long term, a deficiency of any vitamin or mineral can cause physical problems and illness. The 'old-fashioned' diseases such as rickets, scurvy and pellagra have largely disappeared in this country due to our normally plentiful diet, but slimmers following drastic diets for long periods often get symptoms of scurvy, such as bleeding gums, and skin complaints associated with lack of vitamin B. Stress, fatigue, sleeplessness and other symptoms that many dieters think of as simply being associated with eating less are just as likely to be associated with the nutritional shortcomings of the diet.

Ironically, some diets also offer too much of certain nutrients, which can also cause problems. Remember the carrot juice diet? Many people suffered from carotene poisoning after trying that one!

So yes, getting all the nutrients you need for health from your diet can be hard. Even a well thought-out diet, if it contains only a few hundred calories, will be hard pushed to meet all your requirements.

High Speed Slimming avoids any chance of a shortfall in nutrients in two ways. Firstly, it is not drastically low in calories and so there is much more 'room for manoeuvre' than on most slimming diets. Most of you will be dieting on 1 000 calories a day or more and on that level you can easily get enough protein and carbohydrate, a little fat and all the vitamin B, C, iron and calcium, and so on, that you need.

Secondly, I spent a long time analysing the menus personally and I know that they contain enough, but not too much, of all the nutrients. The calories are used to maximum nutritional benefit – not frittered away. There is no danger at all that you will be missing out on anything you need for good health or well-being – that's a promise.

'Fast weight loss will cause me to lose too much lean muscle tissue.'

When you diet, the body doesn't just lose fat but also other matter, including a certain amount of lean body tissue – muscle. In the early '80s it was reported (notably in the RCPh obesity report) that losing weight fast resulted in greater lean tissue loss than slow weight loss, and this was considered a potential health hazard. Several different recent research trials have come to a different conclusion.

Firstly in 1989 the leading publication the *International Journal of Obesity* published the findings of the Howard Research Foundation who tested two groups of overweight females, the first on a diet of 405 calories a day, the second on 800 calories a day, for eight weeks. The ratio of fat-free mass (lean tissue) in the group on the 405 calorie diet fell from 23.0 to 21.3 – not excessive – while the group on 800 calories a day had dropped only from 22.5 to 22.1.

This research study concluded that 'there is no evidence to support the concern that … a rapid rate of weight loss is associated with a disproportionate loss of … lean tissue. No benefit can be demonstrated from restricting rates of weight loss to 1 kg (2.2 lbs) a week.'

Then in 1990 the UK's foremost obesity research centre, the Dunn Clinical Nutrition Centre in Cambridge, carried out a study on seven obese women over a period of 18 weeks, during which time they dieted on as little as 445 calories a day for two weeks at a time, followed by four weeks of eating normally then another two weeks back on the diet, and so on. At the end of the 18-week period an average of 11.25 lbs/5.11 kg had been lost by the women, 82% of which was body fat. The protein (lean body tissue) loss was 0.5 lb/0.25 kg only.

The above experiments were conducted on women who were moderately to severely overweight. A third test was carried out on less overweight women, who needed to lose only a stone or so. Reported in the *IJO* in 1989, the study compared the lean tissue composition of 39 dieters after 8 weeks' dieting against 18 women (of comparable weights to the dieters' *finishing* weights) who had never needed to diet. This study showed an almost identical percentage of fat-free mass between the two groups – 75% for the dieting women and 75.1% for the non-dieting women.

In 1991 the results of multi-centred trials by the Universities of Swansea, Cambridge and Liverpool were reported. When eleven volunteers lost an average of 35.27 lbs/16 kg over a 10-week dieting period, it was found that a minimal 4.75% of the weight lost was protein.

In 1990 over 500 volunteers on diets ranging from 330 to 1500 calories a day were tested at Cambridge University. They dieted continuously from periods of 7 days to 26 weeks and the dieting periods were broken up with unrestricted eating periods which varied in length. The trials established that 'within each person the relative proportion of fat and lean of the weight gained or lost remained the same, regardless of calorie content of the diet ...'

The report went on to conclude that 'nutritionally complete very low-calorie diets do not lead to greater loss of excess lean body tissue than higher-calorie diets.'

But the results of this trial did show that whether weight is lost or gained, every individual has a unique personal ratio of fat to lean within the changed body weight. It now seems that the amount of lean tissue you lose on your diet depends not upon the nature or calorie content of the diet, but upon your own genes.

What is certain is that if you lose weight, you will lose some lean tissue. How much depends on your own make-up – but this loss will be in proportion to fat tissue lost and will be no greater whether you lose 1 lb/450g a week or 5 lbs/2.2 kg a week.

The level of lean tissue loss on *High Speed Slimming* will be kept to a minimum for *you* by containing more than adequate amounts of protein (never less than 20% of total calories) and by a daily programme of muscle-building exercise.

'Dieting slows down your metabolic rate and eventually can make you FAT!'

The book *Dieting Makes You Fat* became a talking point in the mid '80s by putting forward the idea that the more often you go on diets, and the lower in calories those diets are, the more your metabolic rate will slow down so that losing weight becomes harder and harder.

This was based on two main ideas – one, that dieting causes the body to lose a lot of lean tissue (see the second criticism) and that as lean tissue is much more metabolically active (it burns up more calories) than fat tissue, the metabolic rate therefore decreases the more you diet. And two, that when you subject the body to a drastic reduction in calories, it has a natural mechanism that causes it to reduce its own metabolic rate to conserve energy and body fat because it thinks it is going to be starved.

Well, this all sounded very plausible – but much research since then has disproved these theories. We dealt with loss of lean tissue in the previous pages and came to the conclusion that lean tissue loss isn't excessive on normal low-calorie diets. And it does now appear that the drop in metabolic rate due to this minimal loss of lean tissue is also minimal or non-existent.

And the 'starvation' theory appears to be flawed too. In 1990 the Dunn Clinical Nutrition Centre published the findings of an experiment in the *Proceedings of the Nutrition Society*, concluding that there was 'no evidence of lower energy expenditure (i.e. reduction in metabolic rate) in post-obese women.'

The trial compared nine women who had lost

weight and whose weights were now stable with nine women who were matched for age and height and who were and always had been lean, and with nine women who were still overweight. 'There were no significant differences between the lean and the post-obese group in any of the variables, including energy expenditure.' In other words, the ex-dieters were still burning up calories at the rate of the slim women who had never dieted.

Another trial at Dunn – this time to see if the metabolic rate was affected by *repeated* periods of dieting – concluded that although the metabolic rate did change, the differences were 'not significant when corrected for body weight'. At the end of an 18-week period of alternate dieting and non-dieting cycles, the actual metabolic rate of the women per kilogramme of body weight had *increased*. 'Our results in this group of obese women do not suggest that repeated short periods of dieting lead to a cumulative decrease in metabolic rate,' the researchers concluded. In fact, they seemed to indicate the reverse!

The truth is that the metabolic rate of someone who loses weight will drop, but not because of the diet itself, rather because the slimmer now has a lighter body. The heavier you are, the higher your metabolic rate will be. And that is just as true if, for example, a person who has weighed nine stone all her life suddenly puts on weight. At, say, 12 stone/ 76 kg, her metabolic rate will be higher – she will use up an extra 200-300 calories a day just because she weighs more. More energy is needed to move the heavier weight around, to replace lost tissue, and so on. With a lower weight, less energy is needed. So, all other things being equal, anyone who loses weight will end up with a lower metabolic rate than when they were fat. If they put back on all the weight they lost, their rate will go back up.

Further research confirms that the lowered metabolic rate is simply a reflection of the lower weight in the ex-dieter. A study at the University of Pennsylvania in 1990, published in the *Journal of the American Medical Association* (*JAMA*) showed that whether people dieted on 1200 calories a day (and lost an average of 22lbs/9.9kg in 16 weeks) or whether they dieted on less than half that amount (and lost 47lbs/21.3kg in 16 weeks), when they began to eat a maintenance diet, their metabolic rates stabilized at around 9% less than they had been when overweight. The conclusion was that the final drop in metabolic rate simply reflected the weight loss.

As the scientists at Dunn say, 'The post-obese have lower absolute energy requirements compared with their obese state because of the change in weight. Many [post-obese] claim that they have to consume a lower energy intake [fewer calories] to maintain the same weight than those who have never been obese. But our results do not support this.' Other trials in the past two years have come to the same conclusion.

What does all this prove? Simply that once you have lost weight *all other factors being equal* you will have to eat less than you did when fat. But, whether you lose weight quickly or slowly, you will be able to eat a normal amount and not have to live on a lifelong diet of 1000 calories a day, as so many ex-slimmers claim they do.

The *High Speed Slimming* system will ensure that you can eat as much as possible for you to maintain your weight loss because its three keys — diet, lifestyle and exercise — are all designed to make *you* burn up your maximum amount of calories. *High Speed Slimming* will *raise* your metabolic rate. In fact if you take heed of all the tips in this book you may well find that at the end of your slimming period, your metabolic rate is actually higher than it was when you were fat!

On *High Speed Slimming* we are *altering* the metabolic equation in *your* body.

**'Rapid dieting brings psychological problems —
boredom, deprivation, social difficulties and more.'**

Yes, I agree that many ill-thought-out diets do cause considerable psychological suffering to the slimmer, which is why so many diets are abandoned after a very short while.

But on the *High Speed Slimming* system, weight loss is achieved without dropping calorie levels too low so that these problems need never be faced.

The diet is tasty and interesting and is high on filling power. Low blood sugar, and the resultant need to binge, won't occur as 'little and often' eating is a key point within the diet. And after the initial weeks on the diet you can indulge in *free* days when you can eat more – perfect for socializing and entertaining.

'Weight lost quickly stands more chance of being put back on – and of coming back quickly.'

I don't doubt that many thousands of dieters who have lost weight quickly have also put it back on quickly. But there is no physical or scientific reason why this should be the case. You have already read my answers to the second and third criticisms, which go a long way to explaining why there is no physical reason that ex-slimmers should put weight back on again.

But interestingly there appear to have been no trials conducted that actually compare groups of ex-dieters who lost weight slowly with similar groups who lost weight quickly.

In the absence of such trials I telephoned Professor Arnold Bender, the world-famous obesity specialist, who confirmed my suspicions. 'There is no evidence at all,' he said, 'that there is any physical reason that people who lose weight quickly should put it back on more quickly – or more frequently – than people who lose weight slowly.'

The subject of weight maintenance is discussed in full in Chapter Seven. But successful maintenance of weight loss on the *High Speed Slimming* system is probably easier than on any other diet in the world as you will be continuing the principles of the meta-bolism-speeding diet, lifestyle tips and exercise plan that form the core of the weight loss plan itself.

'Crash diets don't re-educate your eating habits.'

That is a very valid criticism. If you spend a few weeks on nothing but milk shakes, or nothing but eggs and grapefruit or carrots and oranges, when 'the diet is finished', what happens next? Firstly, you are so glad to be off the regime that you are likely to binge on anything in sight. And secondly, even if you don't do that, you never want to look at a milk shake (or egg or orange, or whatever) again, so what *can* you eat? Fad diets don't give you a clue as to what should happen next – and if you were overweight in the first place because you hadn't much of an idea about balanced, healthy eating, why should you be any wiser now?

But on *High Speed Slimming* you are retraining your eating habits while you slim down – the diet is based on principles that you can follow healthily and slimly for the rest of your life. And the maintenance chapter will give you all the further help you need.

Well, I think that covers all the criticisms and doubts people have about quick weight loss. So now we can get on with the fun – in the next chapter I'm going to let you into all the secrets of how you're going to get down to target weight – fast!

CHAPTER THREE

The Secret of
High Speed Slimming

The *High Speed Slimming* system is far more than just a reduced-calorie diet. Not only does it never involve a diet of less than 800 calories a day (and the normal for most people is much more than that) but it is a total, four-sided concept for maximum weight loss in minimum time.

This chapter explains in detail how the system works.

EVERYONE IS DIFFERENT

Because I know that different people need different calorie levels, I have devised a system that puts *you* on the right level for *you*.

Why do people vary so much in their calorie needs? People's natural metabolism – the rate at which they use up the calories in their food – varies tremendously depending upon certain factors. Some of those factors we can change (as you will see later). Others we can do little about. And it is these 'fixed factors' that determine your starting calorie level. Let's see what those fixed factors are now.

Age Imagine two women both of the same height, both of the same weight and both similarly active. One burns up 300 calories a day less than the other. Why? Because the one who burns less is aged 60; the one who burns more is aged 30.

For every five years over the age of 25 you are, you burn up approximately 50 calories less a day. Which is why so many people get 'middle-age spread'.

Height The taller you are, the higher your metabolic rate is likely to be, which is why it is sad but true that a woman of 5 ft 6 in can eat far more than a woman of, say, 5 ft 0 in without putting on weight, even if other factors, such as age and fitness levels, are the same.

Body type Some people genetically tend towards a higher rate of metabolism than others. This is largely hereditary and is probably linked to your 'body type'.

There are three types classified. The *ectomorph* type is naturally narrow of build, often with long limbs, has a high metabolic rate and a 'fidgety' mentality – ectomorphs are those lucky people who can eat like horses and still stay slim. They have a high ratio of lean to fat in their bodies – and they probably won't be reading this book.

Then there are the *endomorphs* – many of whom *will* be reading this. You have a high proportion of adipose (fat) tissue: you tend towards soft curves rather than angles and you are the 'cuddly' type, even if you are within the right weight range for your height. As fat burns calories slower than lean tissue, you have a slower metabolic rate than your ecto-morph friend of the same height.

Lastly we have *mesomorphs*, who have a more muscular, 'stocky' frame. If you are naturally meso-morphic, you may weigh the same or more than the endomorph, but you *look* leaner because you have a higher proportion of lean tissue to fat. And you are probably good at many sports and enjoy exercise. You are likely to have a relatively high metabolic rate because lean tissue is much more metabolically active than fat tissue.

Not everyone fits perfectly into one of those three descriptions – most people are a mix of at least two types. But, again, most people can see more of one type in themselves than the other two.

Although you can't alter your basic bone struc-ture or the genes you were born with, you can, with the clever use of exercise, help your body towards what I consider the ideal – the mesomorph type, not too skinny, but with plenty of lean body tissue to burn those calories up quickly.

Sex Males are usually much better at burning up calories than females. This is because women nat-urally tend to be endomorph types with less lean tissue than the average man – though of course there are many exceptions. And women are on average a lot shorter than men. But normally, a man of the same age, height and weight as a woman will have a higher metabolic rate.

Your weight I must have heard hundreds of very overweight people tell me that the reason they are fat is that they have a slow metabolism – they hardly eat a thing yet keep gaining weight (or can't lose it). I am sorry to say that this is a wonderful excuse – but that in 99 cases out of 100, it is simply not true.

The truth is that fat people have a *higher* metabolic rate than slim people, and that, all other things being equal (as we saw in Chapter Two), the slimmer a fat person gets, the slower his or her metabolism will get too, in ratio. One of the main reasons for this is that it takes much more energy (calories) to lift around a 16 stone/101.6 kg body than it does a 10 stone/63.5 kg body. And because even fat people have more lean tissue in their bodies than thin people. It's not quite as simple as that – but almost.

A study conducted by the Dunn Centre proved once and for all that fat people burn up more calories than thin people by measuring accurately the amount of calories fat people consumed. Previous studies had relied on the fat people's own records of what they ate every day, which had seemed to show that indeed they didn't eat more than thin people, and therefore must have slow metabolisms. But in the new study, Dunn found that the fat people's own estimations were, on average, 833 calories *lower* than the truth.

In other words, they ate a lot more than they thought they did!

So if you are starting out very overweight, you can eat hundreds more calories than someone starting out on a diet with only a stone or less to lose, and still lose weight just as quickly – more quickly, probably. Hence there is absolutely no need for anyone with a big weight problem to think that they have to starve to lose weight – they don't.

So all these fixed factors – age, height, body type, sex and starting weight – either increase or decrease the speed at which you burn up calories and influence the speed at which you lose weight. Most people will have some factors in their favour and some against. If you're very lucky you'll have everything going for you and be able to diet easily on a relatively high number of calories – 1500 or so. If you are unlucky and all the fixed factors work against you, you may have to start your diet on a relatively low number of calories – 1000 or so. But even if your fixed factor profile is poor, don't despair because as you'll see, the *High Speed Slimming* system does everything in its power to help you burn off calories faster than ever before.

It is important to know your personal metabolism profile before you start to diet, which is why I have devised a simple questionnaire which *everyone* must do before beginning to slim.

This questionnaire determines *your* correct calorie starting level – which is the *lowest safe level* for you ─ and the *highest level* at which you will lose weight quickly.

The questionnaire is at the start of the next chapter. Don't ignore it ─ it is vital to the success of your slimming campaign.

A UNIQUE, METABOLISM-SPEEDING DIET

The diet, which is the centre of your slimming campaign, uses every calorie-burning technique known to me and, as far as I am aware, is the first diet ever to incorporate all these weight-loss boosting techniques and produce quick loss without starvation-level calories.

Let's run through all the different ways that the *High Speed Slimming* diet does this:

The 60-20-20 balance

The average Western diet contains at least 35% fat, up to 25% protein and up to 40% carbohydrate (much of which is made up of refined and sugary carbohydrates).

The *High Speed Slimming* diet has a different balance. It is 60% carbohydrates, 20% protein and 20% fat. And the carbohydrate content is mostly 'complex' carbohydrates ─ unrefined and natural carbohydrates such as root vegetables, grains, pulses, brown rice and pasta as well as fresh fruits and vegetables. This new balance is not only much health-ier than the average diet — it is also much more effi-cient at slimming you down.

It is the complex carbohydrates that seem more able to convert themselves into energy in your body rather than turning to fat. In other words, a diet high in complex carbohydrates actually speeds up the metabolic rate. And it also appears that a diet high in fat has the opposite effect — it slows it down. As an extreme example, if you ate a diet that was 1000 calories a day of fat, you would lose weight at a much slower rate than if you ate a diet that was 1000 calories a day of carbohydrates.

The most recent study showing this effect was conducted by scientists at Cornell University, New York. The women dieters in the experiment didn't count calories but followed a fairly low-fat (25%) diet, eating as much carbohydrate as they liked. They lost weight slowly but, even more interestingly, their meta-bolic rates *didn't* drop, as would normally be the case with loss of weight (see Chapter Two). The professor in charge of the trials concluded that 'metabolism regulatory mechanisms are related to carbohydrate consumption, not fat.'

The women in the high-carbohydrate experi-ment lost an average of half a pound a week without dieting — and as, theoretically, half a pound of weight lost is equivalent to a calorie burn-off of 1750, that means the high-carbohydrate diet was burning up 1750 ÷ 7 = 250 extra calories a day!

Two years before the New York experiment, *Slimming Magazine* devised a very high-carbohydrate diet (70% of total calories) for its readers who had achieved poor weight losses on conventional diets. Dieting on as much as 1250 calories a day they lost up to 10 lbs in two weeks.

So, clearly, a diet both high in complex carbohydrates and low in fat will work to speed up weight loss for even the most stubborn body. On *High Speed Slimming* we have no need to raise the carbohydrate intake as high as 70% because so many other factors are involved in speeding up your rate of weight loss. And in my own tests I have found that a diet as high as 70% carbohydrate is unpalatable for many people.

I have found that a 60% carbohydrate diet is the ideal compromise, with 20% protein and 20% fat. Any less than 20% protein might deplete the dieter's lean tissue because of the demands of the *High Speed Slimming* exercise programme. And I include 20% fat because this is high enough to make the diet palatable and interesting and yet low enough (lower than the USA trial, you note) to produce the fast slimming effect we want.

As a bonus, the 60-20-20 balance is very high on filling power and is virtually guaranteed to put an end to hunger and food cravings.

The 'little and often' principle

The *High Speed Slimming* diet asks you to eat six

times a day! It is a fact that the act of eating actually speeds up your metabolism. If, for example, you eat 2000 worth of calories a day consisting of six small meals, you will burn up an extra 60-100 calories, whereas if you ate 2000 calories worth of food as two big meals, the burn-up effect would reduce to 20-30 calories.

In other words, on a 'snacking' diet, you can eat more and lose weight just as fast – or perhaps eat the same and lose weight faster.

The snacking principle works because it takes energy to convert food into fuel for the body – and energy is calories burnt. So keep your digestive system working as often as possible and you'll burn off calories with no effort at all. As a good side effect of the snacking system, you will also find that any minor digestive problems will probably disappear. Our systems find it much easier to cope with food received little and often than with nothing to do all day then one big blow-out meal!

You should also eat slowly and chew thoroughly.

'Breakfast like a king …'

Whoever it was who said, 'breakfast like a king, lunch like a prince and dine like a pauper' wasn't far off the mark in dieting terms. On *High Speed Slimming* you won't be eating too many of your calories in the evening although – don't worry! – you *will* be eating *twice* in the evening. The *High Speed Slimming* system spreads the calories out well throughout the day – but ensures that you will be eating most when you are going to burn the food off with exercise before it gets a chance to turn into fat! Most people who tend to eat a main meal late in the evening then do nothing afterwards other than watch TV or go to bed.

The increased metabolic effect of this way of eating is small – but the real advantage is that if you exercise fairly soon after a snack you burn up more calories doing the exercise than you would have had you eaten nothing. The exercise programmes in Chapter Six take advantage of this fact.

Raw food, cool food

You will be eating lots of raw foods and cold foods on the *High Speed Slimming* diet. A hot meal, on average, provides your body with an extra 6 calories of energy more than a similar calorie-value cold meal. So if in theory you ate six hot meals a day you would be adding another 36 calories to your energy intake. By eating most of your meals cold, you don't.

That is only a small saving – but eating cold and raw has another advantage – raw, natural foods such as fruit and salads pass slowly through your stomach and intestines, keeping hunger at bay. But because of their high fibre content, they pass quickly through the bowels, preventing constipation – a complaint suffered by so many people who follow diets other than *High Speed Slimming*.

High C

The diet is high in vitamin C which is known to speed up the metabolic rate as well as enhancing the absorption of vital nutrients such as iron and zinc, to help you feel energetic and keep you healthy while you slim.

And lastly, I have also included plenty of spicy dishes in the menus and recipes – most of which are optional for spice-haters! – because, although I have found no other research confirming their findings, *Slimming* magazine claims that a diet high in chilli and mustard also speeds up metabolic rate by as much as 50% after a meal containing either spice.

And although adding a pinch of chilli or a teaspoon of mustard to your diet may not make much difference to your metabolism, it *will* add a lot of flavour and interest. I prefer the more subtle taste of Dijon mustard to the tongue-numbing English version, but that is up to you. Anyway, I am sure that you will enjoy the international flavour of many of the meal suggestions and recipes in the *High Speed Slimming* diet. From Chicken Tacos to Spicy Satay Sticks – the diet is never boring!

EXTRA CALORIE BURN-UP EFFECT OF HIGH SPEED SLIMMING DIET

By following the high calorie-burning *High Speed Slimming* diet you will be burning up many calories more than if you followed an ordinary diet of the same number of calories. These figures are approximate and vary from person to person. The heavier you are, the greater the extra calorie burn-up is likely to be. The figures given are my estimate of the maximums, which may be added together to give a total maximum potential increase in calorie burn-up effect.

Diet device	Approx. maximum extra calories burnt
Snacking on 6 meals a day	100
Diet high in complex carbohydrates	250
Eating earlier in the day followed by exercise*	25
Eating raw and cold foods	25
Eating vitamin C-rich and spicy foods	25
Total maximum potential increase	425 cals per day

*Calories used in the exercise itself not included in this calculation.

EVERYDAY TECHNIQUES TO ENHANCE YOUR METABOLIC RATE

By using all the tips that follow you could burn off many extra calories every day of your life, in addition to those you are burning off following the *High Speed Slimming* diet and exercise plans. So read these hints carefully and incorporate as many of them as you can into your lifestyle now.

Body consciousness

Fidgety people burn up many more calories a day than tranquil people. That is not to say that I recommend you turn from a calm person into a nervous wreck all for the sake of your waistline – but it *is* worth bearing in mind that a quiet, still body only uses calories at the resting metabolic rate level. The RMR is simply the number of calories you use up per day doing absolutely nothing – i.e. if you just lie asleep for 24 hours. Lying in bed awake uses up hardly any more calories than lying asleep and sitting still in a chair uses up only an extra half a calorie a minute – that's an extra 30 calories an hour – more than you would lying asleep.

But if you sit and fidget you use up many more calories. If you're so fidgety you can't even sit down but pace around the room you'll use an extra 4 or 5 calories a minute. If you stand and do some ironing instead you'll still burn off double what you would have done just sitting there!

It is calculated that most people use only an extra 40% or so calories a day on top of their RMR. So for instance, if a woman's RMR is 1 300 calories a day (fairly average), and she is active at 'average' level, she will use only an extra 520 calories a day, bringing her daily total calorie expenditure to 1820. If such an inactive woman could just raise her activity even 10%, that would mean burning off an extra 130 calories a day.

If you can get the fidget habit – never sitting when you can stand, never standing when you can move, and so on, you could easily raise your own activity level by 10% and see a big difference to how well your diet works.

The fidget also tends to 'bustle around', putting more energy into each movement – whether it's drying a cup or bending down to get something out of a cupboard. Think 'slow' and you think 'slow metabolism'; think 'lively' and you will automatically burn up more calories.

Dash upstairs, don't plod! Hurry to answer the phone, don't dawdle. Knit or sew while you watch TV. You'll not only burn up masses of extra calories a day, you'll be improving your fitness level, too.

Sleep – are you getting too much?

Although the average amount of sleep we are supposed to need a night is eight hours, many people don't need that much, and many more people spend a lot more time in bed than they need to. I know lots of people who lie in a half-sleep for an hour or more every morning, and then take hours longer to feel really awake even when they *do* get up.

I'd start thinking very carefully now about how much time you really do need to spend · in bed, because too much sleep and bed rest is just as bad for you in a different way as too little sleep. If you habitually lie in bed longer than you need, your body will gradually adapt – your body clock will slow down.

So if you take plenty of sleep but still feel sluggish in the mornings for some time after getting up, think about gradually cutting *down* on the amount of time you spend in bed, instead of thinking that perhaps you are *still* not getting enough sleep. At least try this for a night or two before dismissing the idea: set your alarm clock an hour earlier than normal, keep a window open all night – and get up the moment the alarm goes off. I can almost guarantee that you will feel better, not worse – and your metabolism will have received a natural boost.

Aside from this, of course, if you are active for an extra hour each day rather than lying in bed you will burn off more calories. Some light housework will burn off 60 more calories than being in bed will.

How do you breathe?

In order to burn up calories, our bodies need oxygen. If you fill your lungs with air, exercising your lungs and heart as you do so (the heart pumps the oxygen round your body in the blood to the muscles and cells that need it) you make it easier for your body to burn calories than if you spend your time taking shallow breaths.

Most people, however, *do* breathe very shallowly,

using only a small percentage of their lung capacity throughout the day. No wonder, then, that when it comes to time to exercise, the lungs and heart don't know what has hit them and they find it impossible to supply the body with the oxygen it needs.

So every day I would like you to get into the habit of taking in plenty of fresh air. When you get up in the morning, do what our parents used to do — stand in front of the open window and *breathe*. You'll need to practise this, going easy at first as you may feel dizzy.

Throughout the day practise breathing a little more deeply than usual until it becomes second nature — and when you are indoors, make sure that you keep plenty of fresh air circulating through the home.

Remember — fires need oxygen to keep them burning, and so do calories.

Are you keeping cool?

When the weather is hot, your body burns up fewer calories than when it is cold. This is because in cold weather your body needs to burn more of its own fuel to maintain its correct temperature.

Of course, in practice, most of us turn the central heating up in the cold weather and wear more clothes. But you can increase your metabolic rate a little by turning the central heating *down* a notch. You'll save money and help your diet! I don't suggest that you sit in a freezing room in the evenings all winter — but just use your common sense and see if you can bear to keep your cool!

The pleasure factor

Are *you* fed up? It appears that being in a state of depression actually slows down your metabolic rate. So if you tend to be depressive — what can you do about it? Dieting itself can make you depressed — luckily *High Speed Slimming* won't as it is high in tryptophan-rich foods such as milk, cheese and pulses that actually help keep you happy by controlling the levels of serotonin in your brain. Exercise is another anti-depressant — it works by releasing endorphins into the body, so the *High Speed Slimming* system helps there, too.

Sunshine is another anti-depressant, so don't forget to catch all the sun you can. And if you think a too-quiet life might be piling on your pounds, try to get more excitement in your life. Hobbies, friends, laughter, fun — remember, every time you have fun, you are doing your metabolism a favour!

EXTRA CALORIE BURN-UP EFFECT OF HIGH-SPEED SLIMMING LIFESTYLE MODIFICATION TECHNIQUES

Lifestyle device	Approx. maximum extra calories burnt
Body consciousness - increased body movement throughout day (the fidget syndrome) calculated at 10% extra output on a RMR of 1300	130
Taking an hour's less sleep a night and replacing it with mild exercise (e.g. light housework) at 1 extra cal per min over RMR	60
10 mins deep breathing	20
Keeping cool	20
Added excitement (e.g. 30 mins laughing with friends)	20
Total maximum potential increase	250

A UNIQUE *AM/PM* EXERCISE PLAN

Exercise is one of the best metabolism-raisers of all, which is why it is the fourth, very important part of the system. Exercise helps in various ways: firstly, it gives your body a sleeker, firmer, slimmer look and a better shape. These benefits will begin to show just days after starting my regular regime. And for people who have a lot of weight to lose, combining exercise with diet reduces the risk of the 'sag effect' – it tightens up the flab that no amount of dieting alone will do.

Secondly, exercise burns up calories while you are doing it. All exercise burns up calories, but some forms of exercise are better at this than others. The best calorie burners are the aerobic forms of exercise – brisk walking, running, swimming, cycling. All these burn up as many as 500 calories an hour, whereas just sitting in a chair will burn up 90 calories or so. And surprisingly, the heavier you are, the *more* calories you burn up doing exercise. This all means that regular daily exercise is a very useful way of losing weight faster than someone who is on the same calorie-controlled diet but who doesn't exercise.

It is also true that you burn off more calories doing the same exercise if you do it fairly soon after eating something. Although it has become virtually one of the ten commandments that you shouldn't exercise straight after a meal, I am not alone in believing that this only applies to *violent* exertion carried out straight after a *big* meal. Dr Laurence Morehouse is a world expert on fitness, founder of the human performance laboratory at the University College of Los Angeles, author of the exercise sections in the *Encyclopaedia Britannica* and of the bestselling book, *Total Fitness*. He explains that people believe that when you eat, blood is drawn into the intestines and that if you exercise soon after eating, the heart is strained because your muscles need blood, too. But he says that once you begin exercising, the circulation to the intestines shuts down and the muscles get the blood they need.

In any case, the meals in *High Speed Slimming* are not huge, and I suggest that you leave your exercising until about 20-30 minutes after finishing your meal if possible. Exercise then and you will certainly be helping your body to burn off maximum calories. However, if you can't exercise 20-30 minutes after a meal – don't worry. Fit it in when you can as you will still be getting the benefit of burning off hundreds of extra calories.

Thirdly, exercise helps raise your metabolic rate on a longer-term basis than just while you are actually doing the exercise. Studies at the Dunn Clinical Nutrition Centre have shown a small but significant increase in metabolic rate in volunteers the day after periods of exercise have been taken, amounting to an average extra calorie burn-up of 74 a day.

This simply means that if you take regular aerobic exercise, your metabolic rate will be permanently raised – how much depends upon your own metabolic profile and how much exercise you do.

Finally, certain types of exercise help to build muscle – lean tissue – and muscle burns up calories much more quickly than fat does. As I explained in Chapter Two, anyone who loses weight will lose a certain amount of lean tissue inevitably, so this lean-tissue-building effect of regular exercise of the right type is very important. The proportion of muscle in your body can make such a difference to your metabolic rate that it is worth taking a closer look at the subject of 'lean tissue'.

Professor John Durnin, whose book *Energy, Work and Leisure* is used by professionals everywhere in the study of diet and exercise and is recognized as the leading work on the subject, calculates that a person's resting metabolic rate (the calories we burn up daily just to stay alive) can be increased by an average of 300 calories daily by altering the body composition from a high proportion of fat to a high proportion of lean, as is shown in the table overleaf.

As an example, if an overweight 12 stone woman with a high proportion of body fat (RMR 1 500) goes on a diet and loses 3 stone but does no exercise, she will weigh 9 stone but will *still* have a relatively high proportion of body fat and her RMR is likely to be as low as 1 100. But should that women undertake a regular exercise programme such as the *High Speed Slimming* AM/PM plans, she would build muscle tissue as she loses weight and at 9 stone could have a high proportion of lean tissue to fat and a RMR of 1 400.

Calculating then, as explained on pages 45-6, that she uses 50% more calories in her new active lifestyle over and above her RMR, she would burn up 2 100 calories a day. And that is *without* taking into consideration the calories burnt during the actual exercise or all the other metabolism-speeding effects of the *High Speed Slimming* system!

RESTING METABOLIC RATES (in calories per day)
A comparison between RMRs of fat and lean people.

WOMEN	9 stone 126 lbs 57.15 kg	10 stone 140 lbs 63.5 kg	11 stone 154 lbs 69.85 kg	12 stone 168 lbs 76.2 kg	13 stone 182 lbs 82.55 kg
Fat	1100	1300	1400	1500	
Average	1250	1450	1550	1650	
Lean	1400	1600	1700	1800	
MEN					
Fat	1450	1550	1650	1850	
Average	1600	1700	1800	1950	
Lean	1750	1850	1950	2100	

No wonder, then, that exercise is so important for you. Let's conclude by calculating approximately how many extra calories the average slimmer could burn up in a day by following the *High Speed Slimming* exercise programme.

EXTRA CALORIE BURN-UP EFFECT OF HIGH SPEED SLIMMING *AM/PM* EXERCISE PLANS

Exercise factor	Approx. average extra calorie burn-up*
20 minutes a day on the AM plan, cals burnt during	80
20 minutes a day on the PM plan, cals burnt during	120
Raised metabolic rate for following 24 hours	20
Raised metabolic rate due to increase in lean body tissue after maximum tissue increase is reached**	300
Total approximate average potential increase	520

*These figures are for a 10 stone woman with a high proportion of body fat at the outset. The figures will vary from person to person according to weight and other metabolic factors.
**It obviously takes time to build up lean tissue through exercise – the metabolic increase effect therefore will build up gradually over the weeks of exercising to this final maximum.

TO SUMMARIZE ...

So, as you've seen throughout this chapter, on *High Speed Slimming* you have the potential to burn up hundreds and hundreds of extra calories, which is why you can eat plenty and still lose weight fast.

Let's see what that maximum burn-up effect could be:

The diet system .... maximum 425
The lifestyle modifications .... maximum 250
The exercise plans .... maximum 520

Total maximum potential calorie burn-up on all areas of the *High Speed Slimming* system is a quite amazing 1195!

I want to stress that this is a maximum, but – believe me – the potential is quite staggering for *every-one*. Even an extra calorie burn-up of *half* that amount would give quicker weight loss – on more food – than you ever dreamed possible!

Let's take a conservative example of a woman of 11 stone/69.8 kg whose RMR is currently 1400 and who has been using up an extra 40% calories a day in living (an average sort of figure). That means she has been using up 1960 calories a day. Because on average you lose 1 lb/450 g body fat for every 3500 calories you lose on a diet, if she followed a normal 1200 calories-a-day diet she would lose only 1.5 lbs/680 g a week. (1960 minus 1200 daily equals a daily deficit of 760, a weekly deficit of 5 320, divided by 3 500 equals 1.52 lb.)

On the *High Speed Slimming* system, she still starts out with an RMR of 1 400 a day, but in addition to her normal 560 extra calories a day in activity, let us say that she burns off another 600 a day on the *High Speed Slimming* system (remember, that's just *half* the maximum potential and so not unlikely). That means in total she is burning up 1 960 plus 600 which equals 2 560. On a 1 200 calories-a-day diet, that gives her a daily deficit of 1 360, a weekly deficit of 9 520 and a weekly weight loss of nearly 3 lbs/1.3 kg!

If, being a little less conservative, we say her maximum extra calorie burn-up is 800 a day and she follows a 1 000 calories-a-day diet, that gives her a further daily deficit of 400, a further weekly deficit of 2 800 calories, bringing a total deficit of 12 320 and a weekly weight loss of over 3.5 lbs/1.5 kg.

That is *not* taking account of the water/glycogen weight loss at the start of her diet – which will shed a further 5 lbs/2.2 kg or so in the first week of the diet. And it is weight that will continue to be shed at this rate, because of the way the *High Speed Slimming* system works. It won't tail off. It will be weight shed quickly right down to target.

If our dieter of 11 stone/69.8 kg wants to lose 2 stone, she will do it in approximately seven weeks using the above calculations – and never going less than 1 000 calories a day!

Fast weight loss from start to finish — and for men the results are likely to be even more spectacular.

CHAPTER FOUR

The High Speed Slimming Diet Plans

There are four basic plans on the *High Speed Slimming* diet, and everyone will begin to slim on either *Plan One* (1 400 calories a day), *Plan Two* (1 200 calories a day) or *Plan Three* (1 000 calories a day). There are also lists of *extras* so that there are actually *eleven* different starting levels from 1 000 up to 1 500.

To discover your correct starting diet, you must do the short questionnaire that follows. *Do not skip this questionnaire* as it is vital to the success of your plan. And *tell the truth* – there is absolutely no point at all in not doing so – it's *your* diet and we need to make your starting level as near perfect for you as possible. So find a pen, answer the questions now and then I'll explain more about the *High Speed Slimming* system.

HEIGHT/WEIGHT CHART FOR WOMEN

Height	Average weight	Acceptable weight range
4 ft 11 ins	104 lbs	94–122 lbs
1.50 m	47.25 kg	42.75–55.5 kg
5 ft 0 ins	107 lbs	96–125 lbs
1.52 m	48.75 kg	44–57 kg
5 ft 1 ins	110 lbs	99–128 lbs
1.55 m	50 kg	45–58 kg
5 ft 2 ins	113 lbs	102–131 lbs
1.57 m	51.5 kg	46.5–59.5 kg
5 ft 3 ins	116 lbs	105–134 lbs
1.60 m	52.75 kg	47.75–61 kg
5 ft 4 ins	120 lbs	108–138 lbs
1.63 m	54.5 kg	49–62.75 kg
5 ft 5 ins	123 lbs	111–142 lbs
1.65 m	56 kg	50.5–64.5 kg
5 ft 6 ins	128 lbs	114–146 lbs
1.68 m	58 kg	52–66 kg
5 ft 7 ins	132 lbs	118–150 lbs
1.70 m	60 kg	54–68 kg
5 ft 8 ins	136 lbs	122–154 lbs
1.73 m	61 kg	55.5–70 kg
5 ft 9 ins	140 lbs	126–158 lbs
1.75 m	63.5 kg	57–72 kg
5 ft 10 ins	144 lbs	130–163 lbs
1.78 m	65.5 kg	59–74 kg
5 ft 11 ins	148 lbs	134–168 lbs
1.80 m	67 kg	61–76 kg

HEIGHT/WEIGHT CHART FOR MEN

Height	Average weight	Acceptable weight range
5 ft 4 ins 1.63 m	130 lbs 59 kg	118–148 lbs 53.5–67 kg
5 ft 5 ins 1.65 m	133 lbs 60.5 kg	121–152 lbs 55–69 kg
5 ft 6 ins 1.68 m	136 lbs 62 kg	124–156 lbs 56.5–71 kg
5 ft 7 ins 1.70 m	140 lbs 63.5 kg	128–161 lbs 58–73 kg
5 ft 8 ins 1.73 m	145 lbs 66 kg	132–166 lbs 60–75.5 kg
5 ft 9 ins 1.75 m	149 lbs 68 kg	136–170 lbs 62–77 kg
5 ft 10 ins 1.78 m	153 lbs 69.5 kg	140–174 lbs 63.5–79 kg
5 ft 11 ins 1.80 m	158 lbs 72 kg	144–179 lbs 65.5–81 kg
6 ft 0 ins 1.83 m	162 lbs 73.5 kg	148–184 lbs 67–84 kg
6 ft 1 ins 1.85 m	166 lbs 75.5 kg	152–189 lbs 69–86 kg
6 ft 2 ins 1.88 m	171 lbs 78 kg	156–194 lbs 71–88 kg
6 ft 3 ins 1.91 m	176 lbs 80 kg	160–199 lbs 73–90 kg
6 ft 4 ins 1.93 m	181 lbs 82 kg	164–204 lbs 75–93 kg

THE QUESTIONNAIRE

1. Your weight: How much weight do you need to lose? (Check height/weight chart on pages 60-61 if you are not sure.)

MEN	score	WOMEN	score
Over 5 stone 70 lbs/31.75 kg	4	Over 4 stone 56 lbs/25.40 kg	4
3–5 stone 42–70 lbs/19.05–31.75 kg	3	3–4 stone 42–56 lbs/19.05–25.40 kg	3
2–3 stone 28–42 lbs/12.70–19.05 kg	2	2–3 stone 28–42 lbs/12.70–19.05 kg	2
1–2 stone 14–28 lbs/6.35–12.70 kg	1	1–2 stone 14–28 lbs/6.35–12.70 kg	1
Under 1 stone 14 lbs/6.35 kg	0	Under 1 stone 14 lbs/6.35 kg	0

Your score for question 1 ....

2. Your height:

	MEN score	WOMEN score
Over 6 ft/1.83 m	8	5
5 ft 10 ins/1.78 m– 6 ft/1.83 m	7	4

5 ft 7 ins/1.70 m– 5 ft 9½ ins/1.77 m	6	3
5 ft 5 ins/1.65 m– 5 ft 6½ ins/1.69 m	5	2
5 ft 2 ins/1.57 m– 5 ft 4½ ins/1.64 m	4	1
Under 5 ft 2 ins/1.57 m	3	0

Your score for question 2 2

3. Your age:

	MEN and WOMEN score
18–25	2.5
26–30	2.0
31–40	1.5
41–50	1.0
51–60	0.5
61 and over	0

Your score for question 3 .... 1.5

4. Body type: Which of the following descriptions most nearly matches your own natural body shape and type?

MEN and WOMEN score

Mesomorph – a tendency
to muscularity, 'stocky'
build   1

1

63

Ectomorph – long, slim arms and legs, 'straight up and down look'   1

Endomorph – tendency to soft roundness, curves without muscle   0

Your score for question 4 .... *1*

5. Your day: How is your working/typical day spent?

	MEN score	WOMEN score
Very active – e.g. professional sportsman, lumberjack	4	3
Active – e.g. PE teacher, bricklayer	3	2
Average – e.g. doing housework, sales assistant	2	1
Sedentary – e.g. cashier, word processor operator, reading or watching TV	1	0

Your score for question 5 .... *1*

6. Leisure: how much time, *outside of working hours or daily routine already covered in question 5*, do you spend a day walking? (This *does* include time spent walking to and from work.)

MEN and **WOMEN** score

One hour or more	1.5
30 minutes–60 minutes	1.0
15–30 minutes	0.5
Less than 15 minutes	0

Your score for question 6 ....

Finally, write down your scores for the six questions here and add them up for your own personal total.

Question 1	....
Question 2	....
Question 3	....
Question 4	....
Question 5	....
Question 6	....
Your total	......

Now check down the table, find your personal score and discover which plan *you* will be starting on.

PERSONAL TOTAL SCORE	STARTING PLAN
0, 0.5, 1	Plan Three
1.5, 2, 2.5	Plan Three *plus* any *one* 50-calorie addition from the list on page 72
3, 3.5, 4, 4.5	Plan Three *plus* any *one* 100-calorie addition from the list on pages 72-3
5, 5.5, 6, 6.5	Plan Three *plus* any *one* of the 150-calorie additions from the list on page 73
7, 7.5, 8, 8.5	Plan Two
9, 9.5, 10, 10.5	Plan Two *plus* any *one* 50-calorie addition from the list on page 72
11, 11.5, 12, 12.5	Plan Two *plus* any *one* of the 100-calorie additions from the list on pages 72-3
13, 13.5, 14, 14.5	Plan Two *plus* any *one* of the 150-calorie additions from the list on page 73
15, 15.5, 16, 16.5	Plan One

17, 17.5, 18, 18.5	Plan One *plus* any *one* 50-calorie addition from the list on page 72
19, 19.5, 20, 20.5, 21	Plan One *plus* any *one* 100-calorie addition from the list on pages 72-3

Plan Three *see* page 102, Plan Two *see* page 89, Plan One *see* page 75.

BEFORE YOU BEGIN

So now you know which plan you can begin *High Speed Slimming* on. But wait a minute! Before you start, there are a few more things you need to know.

How much weight will I lose?

In the first week of your diet you will lose much more weight than in any other week. More than half of this weight will not be fat, but a combination of glycogen (glucose stored in the muscles and liver) and water. If you lose, for example, 8 lbs in the first week, 4–5 lbs of that will be glycogen and water. This glycogen and water loss slows down during the second week so that gradually the weight loss registering on the scales will be fat (and a small amount of other body tissue) and little else. So don't despair if your first week's weight loss doesn't continue at such a drastic level – it is impossible.

What we are looking for is an average weight loss for you, after the first two weeks or so, of at least 3 lbs a week. For people with a lot of weight to lose the figure is likely to be higher than that but I can't be absolutely precise — I can't say *exactly* how much weight you will lose a week as everyone is different and it depends on how many of the metabolism-boosting effects outlined in Chapter Three you try as well as other factors.

One thing I do know — the *High Speed Slimming* system will lose you *more* weight than you have found possible on other diets of a similar calorie count. Even as you are nearing your target, you should be able to maintain a good weight loss easily. Which brings us to the next question.

How long should I stay on my starting plan?

As long as you are continuing to lose weight at a rate that satisfies you then you can stay on your starting plan for as long as you like. You may find that you can stay on it right down to your target weight, especially if you are doing all the activities recommended in Chapter Six.

However, if your weight loss slows down to below what you consider an acceptable level — say, 3 lbs a week — then all you do is simply move on to the next level. For instance, if you scored 15 in the questionnaire and began dieting on *Plan One* you move on to *Plan Two*, which is 200 calories a day less. If weight loss eventually slows down on that plan too, you move on to *Plan Three*, which is a further 200 calories a day less.

If you were one of the dieters allowed additions on your first plan, you can also have those additions on subsequent plans. Say, if you scored 11 and started dieting on *Plan Two* plus 100 calories, when you move to *Plan Three* you will also be allowed additions worth 100 calories.

What is Plan Four for?

Most people on the *High Speed Slimming* system will find that they easily reach target weight without going lower in calories than *Plan Three*. If you have been on *Plan Three* with either 50-, 100- or 150-calorie additions, and your weight loss slows down, the first thing to do is dispense with the additions and simply follow the basic plan, which is 1000 calories a day. However, some people who scored less than 7 in the questionnaire and *began* dieting on *Plan Three* may find that, towards the end of their diet, they need something a little lower. This is where Plan Four comes in. It is only 800 calories a day and is the plan designed *only* to get those last few pounds off.

No-one should *begin* dieting on Plan Four. And no-one should use Plan Four until their weight loss has slowed down below an acceptable level on Plan Three. Okay?

What if I lose weight too *fast* on my plan?

As I said, filling in the questionnaire should make sure that you start on the plan that is right for you with weight loss that is neither too slow nor too fast. However, there may be exceptions and if you find, after the initial week or two, when you are losing fluid as well as fat (see page 67), that you are losing weight at more than 4 lbs a week or so, then you should increase the calorie level of your diet.

You can do this either by moving back a plan (i.e. from Plan Three to Plan Two or from Plan Two to Plan One) or, if you are on a basic plan with no additions, you can add additions from the lists of up to 150 calories a day. When your weight loss stabilizes at a level with which you are happy, stay there until the loss slows down again and then go back to your original level.

The last alternative is to incorporate a *free day* into your dieting pattern.

This is simply a normal dieting day with up to 400 calories' worth of additions which you are allowed *once a week only*.

However, don't attempt to use the free day concept until you have been dieting for at least four weeks.

THE FREE DAY CONCEPT

The 'free day' can also be used after the first four weeks of dieting to help you over those 'difficult' dieting days – when you want to eat with friends, for example, or when you have a business lunch. All you do is follow the diet for as much of the day as you can, but don't feel guilty about leaving the diet for a few hours to eat what is available. If you follow this free day principle, say, once a fortnight, I estimate that it will make very little difference to your weekly weight loss.

The free day concept is particularly useful for long-term slimmers. I would also like to point out that I know that nearly everyone on a diet eats something they feel they shouldn't have done at some stage – and if they feel bad about it, they are most likely to break the diet completely. So if this happens to you, treat the lapse as a free day and carry on as normal next day.

It will also help if you can increase the amount of exercise you do on your free day, too. For example, do two sessions of the AM plan rather than one, or do some additional activity such as dancing, or make your PM plan thirty minutes instead of twenty. Every little helps!

ADDITIONS

These additions can be made to most of the basic plans as instructed on pages 66-7. Eat them anytime you like during the day.

50-calorie additions

1 piece of fresh fruit, except banana
5 oz/150 g soft fruit of choice
1 diet fruit fromage frais
1 diet fruit yogurt
1½ oz/40 g dried 'no need to soak' apricots or peaches
5 fl oz/140 ml skimmed milk
5 fl oz/140 ml unsweetened orange juice
1 slice wholemeal low calorie bread, e.g. Nimble
2 rye crispbreads
1 oatcake

100-calorie additions

Any *two* additions from 50-calorie list
1 large banana
1½ oz/40 g slice wholemeal bread (average slice from large loaf)
4 oz/100 g potato cooked without fat
1 French-style set fruit yogurt
4½ oz/125 g baked beans in tomato sauce
1 can any WeightWatchers low-calorie soup

5 fl oz/140 ml tub natural low-fat yogurt
4½ oz/125 g tub natural cottage cheese

150-calorie additions

Any *three* additions from 50-calorie list

Any *one* addition from 50-calorie list *plus* any *one*
   addition from 100-calorie list

5 oz/150 g baked potato

1 average wholemeal roll with scraping low-fat
   spread

1 fruit yogurt

1 oz/25 g 'no added sugar' muesli with 4 fl oz/100 ml
   skimmed milk

11 oz/300 g can lentil soup

DAILY ALLOWANCES AND FREE FOODS

Applicable to all plans.

- Daily milk allowance of ¼ pint/140 ml skimmed
milk for use in drinks or on its own. If not used, you
should have one tub of diet fruit yogurt (e.g. Shape)
instead, or one tub of diet fromage frais.
- Unlimited on the diet are weak black tea or coffee
(or with milk from allowance), water, maximum one
fizzy calorie-free diet drink a day, lemon juice, fresh or
dried herbs and spices, green salad leaves. Add
mustard or chilli sauce to any meal you like.

NOTES FOR ALL PLANS

• Try your best to stick to the three meals/three snacks-a-day routine, at intervals of $2\frac{1}{2}$ hours throughout the day. The ideal times are 8.00 AM, 10.30 AM, 1.00 PM, 3.30 PM, 6.00 PM and 8.30 PM. Any allowed additions can be eaten whenever you like.

• For many recipe dishes, alternative, easy-to-prepare meals are given.

• Occasionally, if you dislike a particular meal mentioned, you can swop it for another meal from the same time-band from another day.

• Many of the cold meals can be packed and taken away with you to eat.

• Try to plan ahead so that you have everything you need for the next few days on the diet. Also batch cook when possible – for instance you will often find that there is a rice dish hot one day and that you also need cold rice the next day.

• Unless otherwise stated, 1 slice wholemeal bread' refers throughout all the diets to one average slice of bread from a medium-cut large sliced loaf.

• All references to oil-free French dressing refer to ready prepared low-calorie French dressings of which a number of brands are available (e.g. Waistline from Crosse & Blackwell).

• Part of the *High Speed Slimming* philosophy is that lunch is the largest meal of the day. But if occasionally you find it more convenient to swop the lunch meal around with the tea meal, you can do so.

PLAN ONE

Don't forget your daily milk allowance and *free* foods (see page 73).

Day 1

Breakfast
1½oz/40g 'no added sugar' muesli with 4floz/ 110ml skimmed milk
1oz/28g dried 'no need to soak' apricots, chopped
1 dessert apple, chopped

Snack
¼ pint/140ml unsweetened orange juice
1 diet fruit yogurt
4 'no need to soak' prunes

Lunch
1 portion Chilli con Carne (see recipe page 131) with 4¼oz/110g (cooked weight) boiled brown rice
Large salad of lettuce, cress and green pepper with oil-free French dressing

Snack
1 slice wholemeal bread with a little low-fat spread

Tea
1 portion Pasta and Tuna Salad (see recipe page 145)
1 banana

Snack
1 can low-calorie soup (e.g. WeightWatchers) of
   choice

Day 2

Breakfast
½ grapefruit
2 Weetabix with skimmed milk to cover
5 prunes

Snack
1 slice wholemeal bread with low-fat spread
2 oz/56 g cottage cheese or skimmed milk soft
   cheese

Lunch
1 portion Vegetable and Lentil Curry (see recipe page
   139)
4½ oz/125 g (cooked weight) boiled brown rice
Tomato salad with oil-free French dressing

Snack
1 banana

Tea
1 portion Spiced Chicken in Tomatoes (see recipe
   page 143)
1 slice wholemeal bread with a little low-fat spread
Green salad
2 oz/56 g grapes or cherries *OR* 1 satsuma

Snack
1 diet fromage frais
1 apple

Day 3

Breakfast
1 average bowlful porridge, made with half skimmed
   milk and half water, with 1 oz/20 g sultanas added
1 apple

Snack
1 slice wholemeal bread with a little low-fat spread
2 teaspoons pure fruit spread

Lunch
1 portion Gazpacho Soup (see recipe page 153) *OR*
   1 low-calorie (e.g. WeightWatchers) soup of
   choice
1 portion Spanish Salad (see recipe page 141) *OR*
   4 oz/100 g peeled prawns with 1 dessertspoon
   reduced-calorie mayonnaise, 1 teaspoon tomato
   purée and dash lemon juice mixed in
1 average wholemeal roll
Green salad (no dressing)

Snack
1 orange
1 diet fromage frais

Tea
1 × 8oz/225g baked potato topped with 1 portion Tomato Sauce (see recipe page 150) plus 1 table-spoon Parmesan cheese

Snack
1 banana

Day 4

Breakfast
1 medium-sized egg, boiled
1 slice wholemeal bread with a little low-fat spread
1 orange

Snack
1 × 5floz/140ml tub natural low-fat yogurt
1½oz/40g dried apricots

Lunch
1 double portion Ratatouille Cheese (see recipe page 137)
Green salad with oil-free French dressing

Snack
1 slice wholemeal bread with a little low-fat spread and Marmite

Tea
1 portion Chicken and Walnut Pasta Salad (see recipe page 146)

or

1 average cooked chicken portion, skin removed
1 slice wholemeal bread with a little low-fat spread
Mixed salad with oil-free French dressing.

Snack
1 apple
1 diet fromage frais

Day 5

Breakfast
As Day 1

Snack
1 diet fruit yogurt
1 banana

Lunch
2 oz/56 g very lean ham
1 portion Peanut Coleslaw (see recipe page 146)
1 slice wholemeal bread with a little low-fat spread

Snack
2 rye crispbreads with 2 oz/56 g cottage cheese

Tea
1 portion Chicken Stir-Fry with Noodles (see recipe
    page 128)

Snack
1 orange
1 diet fromage frais

Day 6

Breakfast
As Day 2

Snack
1 slice wholemeal bread with a little low-fat spread
   and 2 teaspoons pure fruit spread
1 satsuma *OR* 2 oz/56 g grapes

Lunch
1 portion Baked Fish with Mustard (see recipe page
   127)
Large portion broccoli
1 × 6 oz/175 g baked potato *OR* 6 oz/175 g boiled
   potatoes

Snack
1 slice wholemeal bread with a little low-fat spread
   and 1 teaspoon honey

Tea
1 portion Spicy Cheese Dip (see recipe page 151)
   with a selection of crudités – raw slices of carrot,
   pepper, radish, spring onion, cauliflower, etc.
1 slice wholemeal toast cut into strips
1 apple

Snack
1 × 5 fl oz/140 ml tub natural low-fat yogurt

Day 7

Breakfast
As Day 3

Snack
1 banana
1 diet fromage frais

Lunch
1 portion Hot Bolognese Mushroom Sauce (see recipe page 149)
5 oz/150 g (cooked weight) boiled wholewheat spaghetti
1 tablespoon grated Parmesan cheese

Snack
1 orange
1 rye crispbread with low-fat spread and Marmite

Tea
1 portion Rice and Smoked Fish Salad (see recipe page 148)
1 small slice wholemeal bread with a little low-fat spread

Snack
1 low-calorie (WeightWatchers) soup of choice

Day 8

Breakfast
As Day 1

Snack
As Day 1

Lunch
1 portion Gazpacho Soup (see recipe page 153)
1 portion Mushroom Risotto (see recipe page 140)

or

1 portion Vegetable and Lentil Lasagne (see recipe
    page 135)
Large mixed salad with oil-free French dressing

Snack
As Day 1

Tea
1 wholemeal pitta bread, split and filled with 1 × 4oz/
    100g can tuna in brine, drained and mixed with
    1oz/28g canned drained butterbeans, 1 chopped
    tomato and 1 spring onion, with oil-free French
    dressing to taste

Snack
1 banana

Day 9

Breakfast
As Day 2

Snack
As Day 2

Lunch
1 large chicken joint, basted with 1 portion Hot
    Barbecue Sauce (see recipe page 150) and grilled
    or baked until cooked
4 oz/100 g (cooked weight) boiled brown rice
Green salad with oil-free French dressing

Snack
1 orange
1 apple

Tea
Sandwich of 2 slices wholemeal bread with a little
    low-fat spread filled with 4 oz/100 g skimmed milk
    soft cheese plus 1 dessertspoon pickle and plenty
    of lettuce, cress, cucumber, 2 sticks celery

Snack
1 low-calorie (WeightWatchers) soup of choice

Day 10

Breakfast
As Day 3

Snack
As Day 3

Lunch
1 portion Liver in Mustard Sauce (see recipe page 132)
5 oz/140 g new potatoes *OR* 4 oz/100 g potato mashed with a little milk from allowance and ¼ oz/7 g low-fat spread
Large serving broccoli or spring greens

Snack
As Day 3

Tea
1 portion Lentil Dip (see recipe page 152)
1 wholewheat pitta bread
Green side salad dressed with lemon juice and black pepper

Snack
1 banana

Day 11

Breakfast
As Day 4

Snack
As Day 4

Lunch
1 portion Seafood Stir-Fry (see recipe page 124)
6oz/175g (cooked weight) boiled brown rice
Mixed side salad with oil-free French dressing

Snack
As Day 4

Tea
1 portion Pasta Salad with Chilli Dressing (see recipe
    page 147) on bed of lettuce

Snack
As Day 4

Day 12

Breakfast
As Day 5

Snack
As Day 5

Lunch
1 double portion Spicy Bean Casserole (see recipe
    page 138)
Green salad with oil-free French dressing

Snack
As Day 5

Tea
4oz/100g peeled prawns and 1 dessertspoon
    reduced-calorie mayonnaise
1 large (2oz/50g) slice wholemeal bread with a little
    low-fat spread
Green salad dressed with lemon juice and black
    pepper

Snack
As Day 5

Day 13

Breakfast
As Day 2

Snack
As Day 6

Lunch
1½oz/40g Parma ham with 1 large slice ripe Ogen
    or Charentais melon and 1 average wholemeal roll

OR sandwich of 2 slices wholemeal bread and a little low-fat spread filled with 2 oz/56 g very lean ham and tomato

either choice followed by

1 banana
1 diet fromage frais

Snack
1 × 5 fl oz/140 ml tub natural low-fat yogurt

Tea
1 portion Cod in Orange Sauce (see recipe page 126) *OR* 1 × 175 g cod steak grilled with 1 slice lemon
5 oz/140 g boiled potatoes
4 oz/100 g carrots
4 oz/100 g French beans

Snack
1 low-calorie (WeightWatchers) soup of choice

Day 14

Breakfast
As Day 3

Snack
As Day 7

Lunch
1 portion Beef Stroganoff (see recipe page 134)
4½oz/125g (cooked weight) boiled brown rice
Green side salad

Snack
As Day 7

Tea
1 portion Egg and Tuna Salad (see recipe page 142)
1 slice wholemeal bread with a little low-fat spread

Snack
1 large slice melon *OR* 4oz/100g grapes
1 diet fruit yogurt

If you wish to continue on *Plan One*, simply repeat as often as necessary starting from Day 1.

For faster weight loss you may move to *Plan Two* as explained at the start of this chapter.

If you have now reached target weight, turn to Chapter Seven.

PLAN TWO

Don't forget your daily milk allowance and *free* foods
(see page 73).

Day 1

Breakfast

1½oz/40g 'no added sugar' muesli with 4floz/
110ml skimmed milk

1oz/28g dried 'no need to soak' apricots, chopped

1 dessert apple, chopped

Snack

1 diet fruit yogurt

1 orange

Lunch

1 portion Vegetable and Lentil Lasagne (see recipe
page 135)

Green salad with oil-free French dressing

Snack

1 banana

Tea

1 medium sized egg *OR* 2oz/56g very lean ham

1 average wholemeal roll with a little low-fat spread

Large salad of cress, lettuce, cucumber, peppers,
tomato and spring onion in oil-free French
dressing

Snack
1 diet fromage frais
1 apple

Day 2

Breakfast
½ grapefruit
2 Weetabix with skimmed milk to cover
5 prunes

Snack
2 rye crispbreads with a little low-fat spread
1 pear or peach

Lunch
1 wholemeal pitta bread split and filled with ½ ×
   6oz/185g can Tuna in Barbecue Sauce (e.g. John
   West) plus chopped cucumber and lettuce
1 satsuma *OR* 3½oz/ 80g grapes

Snack
1 diet fromage frais
1½oz/40g dried apricots

Tea
1 portion Ratatouille Cheese (see recipe page 137)
1 small slice wholemeal bread

Snack
1 apple
1 orange

Day 3

Breakfast

1 average bowlful porridge, made with half skimmed milk and half water, with 1 oz/20 g sultanas added

1 apple

Snack

1 diet fruit yogurt

1 orange

Lunch

1 large cooked chicken joint, skin removed

1 average wholemeal roll

Mixed salad with oil-free French dressing

Snack

1 banana

Tea

1 portion Cod in Orange Sauce (see recipe page 126) *OR* 7 oz/200 g cod steak grilled with lemon juice

4 oz/100 g new potatoes

4 oz/100 g green beans

Snack

1 low-calorie (WeightWatchers) soup of choice

Day 4

Breakfast
1 medium-sized egg, boiled
1 slice wholemeal bread with a little low-fat spread
1 orange

Snack
1 diet fruit yogurt
1½oz/40g dried apricots

Lunch
1 portion Chilli con Carne (see recipe page 131)
4oz/100g (cooked weight) boiled brown rice

or

Sandwich of 2 slices wholemeal bread with a little
  low-fat spread, filled with 3oz/80g very lean roast
  beef, horseradish and green salad items
1 apple

Snack
1 slice wholemeal bread with a little low-fat spread
  and Marmite

Tea
1 × 4¼oz/110g VegeBurger (from dry mix pack
  available in health food stores and supermarkets
  or frozen ready-made), grilled
Tomato and onion salad in oil-free French dressing
Small slice wholemeal bread

Snack
1 apple
1 pear

Day 5

Breakfast
As Day 1

Snack
1 diet fruit yogurt
1 orange

Lunch
1 portion Spanish Salad (see recipe page 141)
4 oz/100 g grapes *OR* 1 pear

Snack
1 slice wholemeal bread with a little low-fat spread
and 1 teaspoon pure fruit spread

Tea
1 × 7 oz/200 g baked potato topped with 1 portion
Tomato Sauce (see recipe page 150)

or

1 × 11 oz/300 g can lentil soup with 1 average
wholemeal roll

Snack
1 diet fromage frais
2 rye crispbreads with a little low-fat spread

Day 6

Breakfast
As Day 2

Snack
1 slice wholemeal bread with a little low-fat spread
and 1 teaspoon honey

Lunch
1 large chicken breast portion, skinned and coated
with 1 portion Hot Barbecue Sauce (see recipe
page 150) and grilled or baked
3 oz/80 g new potatoes
Green salad with oil-free French dressing

Snack
1 banana

Tea
1 portion Pasta and Tuna Salad (see recipe page
145)
1 small slice wholemeal bread

Snack
1 apple
1 diet fruit yogurt

Day 7

Breakfast
As Day 3

Snack
1 diet fromage frais
1 orange

Lunch
1 portion Hot Bolognese Mushroom Sauce (see recipe page 149)

1 × 6oz/175g baked potato *OR* 5oz/150g (cooked weight) boiled wholewheat pasta of choice

Snack
1 slice wholemeal bread with a little low-fat spread and Marmite

Tea
Sandwich of 2 slices wholemeal bread with a little low-fat spread, filled with 4oz/100g skimmed milk soft cheese plus 1 dessertspoon piccalilli and 1 tomato

Snack
1 banana

Day 8

Breakfast
As Day 1

Snack
As Day 1

Lunch
1 portion Liver in Mustard Sauce (see recipe page 132)
4oz/100g French beans or broccoli
2½oz/70g new potatoes

Snack
As Day 1

Tea
1 × 6oz/175g baked potato topped with a *half* portion Chilli con Carne (see recipe page 131)
Green salad

Snack
1 apple

Day 9

Breakfast
As Day 2

Snack
As Day 2

Lunch
1 portion Seafood Stir-Fry (see recipe page 124)
4 1/2 oz/140 g (cooked weight) boiled brown rice
Salad of tomato, onion, and watercress with oil-free
    French dressing

Snack
As Day 2

Tea
1 wholemeal pitta bread split and filled with 3 oz/80 g
    cottage cheese, pinch chilli powder and chopped
    tomato, cucumber and pepper

Snack
As Day 2

Day 10

Breakfast
As Day 3

Snack
As Day 3

Lunch
1 portion Spicy Bean Casserole (see recipe page
    138)
1 average wholemeal roll

Snack
As Day 3

Tea
1 portion Egg and Tuna Salad (see recipe page 142)
2 rye crispbreads with low-fat spread

Snack
As Day 3

Day 11

Breakfast
As Day 4

Snack
As Day 4

Lunch
1 portion Tomato Sauce (see recipe page 150) on
    6oz/175g (cooked weight) boiled wholewheat
    pasta of choice, topped with 1 tablespoon grated
    Parmesan cheese
Green salad with oil-free French dressing

Snack
As Day 4

Tea
1 portion Tabbouleh (see recipe page 144)
1 apple

Snack
1 banana

Day 12

Breakfast
As Day 1

Snack
As Day 5

Lunch
1 portion Baked Fish with Mustard (see recipe page 127)
4½oz/140g baked potato
Large mixed salad with oil-free French dressing

Snack
As Day 5

Tea
Sandwich of 2 slices wholemeal bread with a little low-fat spread, filled with 2oz/56g very lean ham and 1 teaspoon mustard
1 tomato

Snack
1 diet fromage frais
1 apple

Day 13

Breakfast
As Day 2

Snack
As Day 6

Lunch
1 portion Chicken and Walnut Pasta Salad (see recipe page 146)
1 orange

Snack
As Day 6

Tea
1 portion Mushroom Risotto (see recipe page 140)

Snack
As Day 6

Day 14

Breakfast
As Day 3

Snack
As Day 7

Lunch
1 portion Beef and Pepper Stir-Fry (see recipe page 133)
Tomato and lettuce salad with oil-free French dressing

Snack
As Day 7

Tea
1 portion Rice and Smoked Fish Salad (see recipe page 148)
1 diet fruit yogurt

Snack
1 banana

If you wish to continue on *Plan Two*, simply repeat as often as necessary starting from Day 1.

For faster weight loss you may move to *Plan Three* as explained at the start of this chapter.

If you have now reached target weight, turn to Chapter Seven.

PLAN THREE

Don't forget your daily milk allowance and *free* foods
(see page 73)

Day 1

Breakfast
1 oz/28 g 'no added sugar' muesli with 4 fl oz/110 ml
    skimmed milk to cover
1 orange

Snack
1 banana

Lunch
1 large egg, hard-boiled *OR* 2 oz/56 g very lean ham
1 portion salad dressing made from 1 dessertspoon
    reduced-calorie mayonnaise and 1 dessertspoon
    natural yogurt mixed with *either* ½ teaspoon curry
    powder *or* paprika *or* mustard
Large salad of green leaves, cucumber, tomato,
    radish
1 slice wholemeal bread with a little low-fat spread

Snack
1 diet fruit yogurt of choice
1 apple

Tea
5 oz/140 g baked beans on 1 slice wholemeal toast
(no butter)

or

1 portion Spicy Bean Casserole (see recipe page
138)

Snack
1 apple

Day 2

Breakfast
½ grapefruit
2 Weetabix with skimmed milk to cover

Snack
2 rye crispbreads with 2 oz/56 g low-fat soft cheese

or

1 oz/28 g hummus
Tomato slices

Lunch
1 wholemeal pitta bread split and filled with ½ ×
6 oz/185 g can Tuna in Barbecue Sauce (e.g. John
West) plus chopped iceberg or any other crisp leaf
lettuce, cucumber and green pepper

or

1 × 3½oz/100g can tuna in brine, drained, with 1 average wholemeal roll and a little low-fat spread
Large mixed salad with oil-free French dressing

Snack
1 apple

Tea
1 portion Ratatouille Cheese (see recipe page 137)

or

1½oz/40g reduced-fat Cheddar-style cheese and 1 sliced tomato melted on 1 slice wholemeal toast

Snack
1 orange

Day 3

Breakfast
1½oz/40g Bran Flakes with skimmed milk to cover

Snack
1 banana

Lunch
1 average cooked chicken portion, skin removed
Green salad
1 average wholemeal roll with a little low-fat spread

Snack
1 nectarine *OR* 3 oz/80 g grapes
1 diet fruit yogurt

Tea
1 portion Chilli King Prawns (see recipe page 123)
Side salad

or

4 oz/110 g peeled prawns dressed with lemon juice
and black pepper on shredded iceberg or any other
crisp leaf lettuce, with 1 slice wholemeal bread and
a little low-fat spread

Snack
1½ oz/40 g 'no need to soak' dried apricots *OR* 1
pear

Day 4

Breakfast
½ grapefruit
1 boiled or poached medium-sized egg
1 slice wholemeal bread

Snack
1 diet fruit yogurt
1 apple

Lunch
1 portion Chilli con Carne (see recipe page 131)
2 tablespoons boiled brown rice
Green salad

or

Sandwich of 2oz/56g very lean ham and mustard in
    2 slices wholemeal bread with as much tomato,
    lettuce and cress as you can cram in
1 diet fruit fromage frais

Snack
1 slice wholemeal bread with Marmite or 1 teaspoon
    honey

Tea
1 × 4oz/110g VegeBurger (from dry mix pack avail-
    able in health food stores and supermarkets or
    frozen ready-made), grilled
Large mixed salad
1 teaspoon tomato relish

Snack
1 orange

Day 5

Breakfast
1oz/28g 'no added sugar' muesli, with skimmed milk
    to cover, plus 1oz/28g dried apricots, peaches *or*
    prunes

Snack
1 dried fruit yogurt
1 orange

Lunch
1 portion Chicken Stir-Fry with Noodles (see recipe
   page 128)

or

Same as Day 3

Snack
1 banana
2 oz/56 g grapes

Tea
1 slice wholemeal bread with 4 oz/113 g cottage
   cheese of choice plus tomato and lettuce

Snack
1 apple

Day 6

Breakfast
As Day 2

or

1/2 grapefruit
1 slice wholemeal toast with a little low-fat spread
   and 2 teaspoons reduced-sugar marmalade or jam

Snack
5 fl oz/150 ml natural yogurt

Lunch
1 portion Spanish Salad (see recipe page 141)

Snack
1 slice wholemeal bread with Marmite

Tea
1 × 6 oz/175 g baked potato with topping of *EITHER*
   2 tablespoons sour cream and chopped chives *OR*
   2 oz/56 g cottage cheese mixed with paprika
Side salad

Snack
1 1/2/40 g dried apricots

Day 7

Breakfast
As Day 3

Snack
1 diet fruit yogurt
1 orange

Lunch
1 portion Vegetable and Lentil Lasagne (see recipe page 135)

or

1 frozen Vegetable Lasagne (e.g. Birds Eye)

Snack
1 banana

Tea
1 portion of Egg and Tuna Salad (see recipe page 142)

Snack
1 apple

Day 8

Breakfast
As Day 1

Snack
As Day 1

Lunch
1 portion Liver in Mustard Sauce (see recipe page 132)
Large serving broccoli or spring greens
2 tablespoons peas

Snack
As Day 1

Tea
1 portion Gazpacho Soup (see recipe page 153)
1 slice wholemeal bread

Snack
As Day 1

Day 9

Breakfast
As Day 2

Snack
As Day 2

Lunch
1 portion Chicken Tacos (see recipe page 129)
Green salad

or

As Day 3

Snack
As Day 2

Tea
2oz/56g feta cheese, crumbled and mixed with

chopped tomato, cucumber, green pepper, onion, lettuce and a couple of black olives and tossed in oil-free French dressing
1 mini pitta

Snack
As Day 2

Day 10

Breakfast
As Day 3

Snack
As Day 3

Lunch
1 portion Vegetable and Lentil Curry (see recipe page 139)
3 tablespoons boiled brown rice

Snack
As Day 3

Tea
1 portion Rice and Smoked Fish Salad (see recipe page 148) served on bed of lettuce

Snack
As Day 3

Day 11

Breakfast
As Day 4

Snack
As Day 4

Lunch
1 portion Seafood Stir-Fry (see recipe page 124)
5 tablespoons boiled brown rice
Green salad

or

Sandwich of 2 slices wholemeal bread with a little low-fat spread, filled with 3½oz/80g peeled prawns and 1 level dessertspoon reduced-calorie mayonnaise plus lettuce and cucumber

Snack
As Day 4

Tea
1 portion Spiced Chicken in Tomatoes (see recipe page 143)
1 rye crispbread with a little low-fat spread
Green salad

Snack
As Day 4

Day 12

Breakfast
As Day 5

Snack
As Day 5

Lunch
1 portion Tuna, Lentil and Rice Stuffed Peppers (see recipe page 125)
2 rye crispbreads with a little low-fat spread

or

As Day 2

Snack
As Day 5

Tea
Selection of crudités – e.g. strips of raw carrot, celery, white cabbage, radish, pepper, cauliflower with 1 portion Spicy Cheese Dip (see recipe page 151)

Snack
As Day 5

Day 13

Breakfast
As Day 6

Snack
As Day 6

Lunch
1 portion Spicy Satay Sticks (see recipe page 130)
Green salad

or

As Day 3

Snack
As Day 6

Tea
1 portion Tabbouleh (see recipe page 144) served on
    green leaves

Snack
As Day 6

Day 14

Breakfast
As Day 3

Snack
As Day 7

Lunch
1 average wholemeal roll with a little low-fat spread
   filled with 2oz/56g reduced-fat Cheddar-style
   cheese plus large mixed salad wtih oil-free French
   dressing

Snack
As Day 7

Tea
1 portion Baked Fish with Mustard (see recipe page
   127)
Green side salad dressed with lemon juice and black
   pepper

Snack
As Day 7

If you wish to continue on *Plan Three*, simply repeat
as often as necessary starting from Day 1.

   If you are near target weight, for faster weight
loss you may move to *Plan Four* after reading the
conditions on page 69 of this chapter.

   If you have now reached target weight, turn to
Chapter Seven.

PLAN FOUR

Don't forget your daily milk allowance and the *free* foods (see page 73).

Use this plan to lose the last few pounds only.

Day 1

Breakfast
1 oz/28 g bran flakes or oatbran flakes with ¼ pint/ 140 ml skimmed milk

Snack
1 banana

Lunch
1 portion Spicy Cheese Dip (see recipe page 151) with a selection of crudites, e.g. slices of raw carrot, pepper, spring onions, cauliflower, radish
1 apple

Snack
1 orange

Tea
5 oz/140 g baked beans on 1 slice wholemeal toast

or

1 portion Spicy Bean Casserole (see recipe page 138)

Snack
1 diet fruit yogurt or fromage frais

Day 2

Breakfast
1 × 5 fl oz/140 ml tub natural low-fat yogurt with
      ½oz/15g 'no added sugar' muesli mixed in

Snack
1 banana

Lunch
1 portion Egg and Tuna Salad (see recipe page 142)

Snack
1 orange

Tea
1 portion Ratatouille Cheese (see recipe page 137)
Green salad with oil-free French dressing

Snack
1 diet fruit yogurt or fromage frais

Day 3

Breakfast
1 × 1½oz/40g slice wholemeal toast with a little
      low-fat spread and 2 teaspoons pure fruit spread

Snack
1 banana

Lunch
1 portion Lentil Dip (see recipe page 152) with
    crudités as Day 1 plus 1 rye crispbread

Snack
1 orange

Tea
1 portion Chilli King Prawns (see recipe page 123)
2 tablespoons boiled brown rice

Snack
1 diet fruit yogurt or fromage frais

Day 4

Breakfast
1 medium-sized egg, boiled
1 × 1 oz/28 g slice wholemeal bread

Snack
1 banana

Lunch
1 portion Rice and Smoked Fish Salad (see recipe
    page 148)

or

1 small can (3½oz/100g) tuna in brine in 2 slices
   low-calorie wholemeal bread (e.g. Nimble) with 1
   sliced tomato

Snack
1 orange

Tea
1 × 4oz/110g VegeBurger (from dry mix pack available in health food stores and supermarkets or
   frozen ready-made), grilled
Mixed salad with oil-free French dressing

Snack
1 diet fruit yogurt or fromage frais

Day 5

Breakfast
As Day 1

Snack
1 banana

Lunch
1 portion Spiced Chicken in Tomatoes (see recipe
   page 143)
1 apple

or

3½oz/100g cooked skinless chicken
Mixed salad with oil-free French dressing
2 rye crispbreads with a little low-fat spread

Snack
1 orange

Tea
1 × 6oz/175g baked potato filled with 2oz/56g cottage cheese and a pinch chilli powder

Snack
1 diet fruit yogurt or fromage frais

Day 6

Breakfast
As Day 2

Snack
1 banana

Lunch
1 portion Pasta and Tuna Salad (see recipe page 145)

Snack
1 orange

Tea
1 × 11oz/300g can lentil soup with 1 × 1oz/28g slice wholemeal bread

Snack
1 diet fruit yogurt or fromage frais

Day 7

Breakfast
As Day 3

Snack
1 banana

Lunch
1 portion Tabbouleh (see recipe page 144)

or

1 medium-sized egg, hard-boiled and sliced in 2 slices of low-calorie wholemeal bread (e.g. Nimble) with 1 sliced tomato

Snack
1 orange

Tea
1 portion Tomato Sauce (see recipe page 150) on 4oz/110g (cooked weight) wholewheat pasta of choice

Snack
1 diet fruit yogurt or fromage frais

Now you are at target weight, turn to Chapter Seven.

CHAPTER FIVE

The High Speed Slimming recipes

The recipes that follow are all used in one or more of the *High Speed Slimming* diets in Chapter Four. The calorie counts given are for the recipes only and don't include any of the accompaniments mentioned within the diets.

All recipes serve *four* but quantities can easily be halved to serve two. Many recipes are suitable for freezing or will keep for several days in the fridge, so if you are on your own it is well worth making up a full quantity of these dishes and saving what you don't use – to save *your* time.

I have chosen only recipes that require no elaborate preparation or lengthy cooking because I know that most high-speed slimmers also lead high-speed lives. This is fast food with a difference and so, even though there are often plainer alternatives to choose within each diet, do give some of these dishes a try as they will add taste and interest to your slimming campaign – two vital factors for success.

Demi-vegetarians will find many suitable recipes here. *Vegetarians* have a selection of main course dishes plus several other suitable dishes in the

Salads and *Dips and Sauces* sections. There are also some suggestions for adapting non-vegetarian recipes to suit vegetarians at the end of several dishes in the *Note* section.

FISH AND SEAFOOD

Chilli King Prawns

155 calories per portion
Not suitable for freezing or storing in fridge

24 king prawns
1 clove garlic, crushed
1 tablespoon tomato
    purée
1 tablespoon red wine
    vinegar
1 dessertspoon
    Worcestershire sauce
1 dessertspoon soya
    sauce

3 level teaspoons sugar
1 dried red chilli,
    de-seeded, crushed
1 red pepper, de-seeded
    and cut into squares
1 dessertspoon cornflour
    blended with
    3 fl oz/75 ml fish stock
    or water

Shell the prawns but leave the tails on. Combine garlic, tomato purée, vinegar, sauces, sugar and chilli in a bowl and add the prawns. Leave in fridge to marinate for an hour or two.

Soak four bamboo sticks or use steel kebab sticks and thread prawns and pepper alternately onto them. Grill or barbecue on a medium heat until prawns are cooked, brushing with the chilli mixture.

To serve, combine cornflour mixture with rest of chilli mixture in small pan and heat, stirring, until sauce thickens.

Note: 500g fillet of monkfish may be substituted for the prawns, in which case the recipe contains 135 calories per portion.

Seafood Stir-Fry

170 calories per portion
Not suitable for freezing or storing in fridge

8oz/225g large peeled prawns, cooked

12oz/325g cubed monkfish (or cod) fillet

6oz/175g button mushrooms, sliced

1 small green pepper, de-seeded and sliced

4 spring onions, chopped

1 dessertspoon corn oil

2 tablespoons dry sherry

little fish or chicken stock from cube

3/4"/2cm piece fresh or dried ginger

2 teaspoons cornflour mixed with a little cold water

1 tablespoon tomato purée

1 tablespoon soya sauce

salt and black pepper

Heat the oil in a wok or non-stick frying pan and add the monkfish cubes, the onions and pepper. Stir fry for a few minutes then add the mushrooms, prawns, sherry, ginger and stir-fry for a couple more minutes, adding a little of the stock if necessary. Lastly add the cornflour mixture, tomato purée, soya sauce and a little more stock, and stir until you have a rich sauce. Taste the sauce and season as necessary.

Note: If using uncooked prawns, add them at the same time as the monkfish.

Tuna, Lentil and Rice Stuffed Peppers

250 calories per portion
Not suitable for freezing but can be stored in fridge for 24 hours

2 large red peppers, halved lengthways and de-seeded
1 medium onion, finely chopped
1 × 14oz/400g can chopped tomatoes
1 × 6½oz/185g can tuna in brine, drained
8oz/225g (cooked weight) boiled brown rice
4oz/110g (cooked weight) boiled brown lentils
1 clove garlic, crushed
1 teaspoon oregano
4 low-fat cheese slices (e.g. Singles) or 2oz/56g sliced mozzarella cheese
1 tablespoon olive oil

Heat the oil in a frying pan and sauté the onion until soft and just turning golden. Add the tomatoes, rice, lentils, garlic and oregano, stir and simmer for a few minutes to thicken. Add tuna and a little seasoning if necessary and divide the stuffing between the peppers.

Bake at 180°C/350°F/Mark 4 for 20 minutes then top each stuffed pepper with a cheese slice and grill under a medium heat until cheese is bubbling.

Note: Brown lentils are quick to cook – just add 18 fl oz/500 ml water for every 4 oz/110 g dry weight lentils and boil for 10 minutes, then simmer for a further 30 minutes or until tender.

Cod in Orange Sauce

140 calories per portion
Can be frozen and reheated in microwave

4 × 6 oz/175 g cod (or other white fish) steaks
4 fl oz/110 ml orange juice
1 tablespoon light soya sauce
½ teaspoon ground ginger or level teaspoon grated fresh ginger
1 heaped teaspoon cornflour blended with a little water or fish stock
1 teaspoon grated orange peel
a little fish stock
orange slices to decorate

Blend orange juice, soya sauce, ginger and orange peel in a bowl and add fish steaks. Leave to marinate for an hour or two then place fish and marinade in a non-stick frying pan and sauté until steaks are cooked.

Remove steaks and keep warm. Add cornflour mixture to pan, stir constantly until sauce thickens, adding a little more fish stock as necessary. Serve with the fish and garnish with orange slices.

Note: Cod steaks work well in this recipe, but plaice, monkfish or halibut are good too.

Baked Fish with Mustard

190 calories per portion
Not suitable for freezing or storing

4 × 7 oz/200 g haddock
   or cod fillets
4 level teaspoons Dijon
   mustard
2 tablespoons lemon
   juice
1 teaspoon lemon rind,
   grated

2 tablespoons fresh
   parsley, chopped
4 oz/110 ml natural
   Greek yogurt
salt and black pepper
1 teaspoon corn oil

Blend together the mustard, lemon juice, rind, half the parsley, the yogurt and seasoning. Cut four oblongs of tinfoil large enough to form a loose parcel round each fillet. Brush each with oil. Place a fillet in the centre of each piece of foil and form an open parcel. Pour a quarter of the sauce into each parcel and seal. Bake at 200°C/400°F/Mark 6 for 20 minutes. Serve in the foil on the plates, handing round the remaining parsley for garnish.

Note: All fish is good cooked *en papillote* (in a parcel). Just add your favourite spices and herbs with a dash of lemon juice or wine for a tasty low-calorie meal.

POULTRY

Chicken Stir-Fry with Noodles

295 calories per portion
Suitable for freezing or to store in fridge for one day

4 × 3½oz/100g boned skinless chicken breast fillets, cut into bite-sized pieces

6oz/175g button mushrooms, sliced

4 spring onions, chopped

4oz/110g fresh beansprouts

1 dessertspoon corn or olive oil

1 clove garlic, crushed

1 small piece fresh or dried ginger

½ teaspoon ground cumin seeds

1 tablespoon oyster sauce

1 heaped teaspoon cornflour blended with a little cold chicken stock from cube

a little chicken stock

4½oz/140g dried noodles, cooked according to packet instructions

Heat the oil in a wok or non-stick frying pan and add

the chicken, stirring, for a few minutes. Add all the rest of the ingredients except the cornflour and noodles and cook for 3 more minutes, stirring all the while. Add a little chicken stock if necessary. Now add the cornflour and a little more chicken stock, allow sauce to bubble and finally add the noodles, stirring just to heat through.

Note: If using cooked chicken, add to pan at the same time as the mushrooms, etc.

Chicken Tacos

300 calories per portion
Not suitable for freezing – chicken filling can be stored in an airtight container in the fridge for a day

8 taco shells
Half an 8 oz/225 g jar
   taco sauce, mild or hot
   to suit taste
8 oz/225 g cooked
   chicken meat, no skin,
   chopped
5 oz/140 g red kidney
   beans, canned
   (drained weight)

8 oz/225 g shredded
   iceberg or any other
   crisp leaf lettuce
4 oz/110 g reduced-fat
   Cheddar-style cheese,
   grated

Heat the chicken, sauce and beans in a saucepan until warm. Warm the taco shells as instructed on packet. Line each shell with some lettuce, top with some of the chicken mixture then the grated cheese and a little more lettuce.

Note: Very lean (less than 10% fat) minced beef or TVP mince could be used in this recipe for a change. Dry-fry the meat in a non-stick pan, stirring, until well brown, then add the sauce and kidney beans and simmer for a few minutes or until beef is tender. Calorie count is the same.

Spicy Satay Sticks

280 calories per portion
For storing instructions see below

1 lb/450 g chicken breast
  or pork fillet, cubed
2 tablespoons Chilli and
  Garlic sauce (e.g. Lea
  & Perrins)
1 teaspoon corn or olive
  oil

For the Sauce:
2½ oz/62.5 g crunchy
  peanut butter
3 fl oz/75 ml water
1 tablespoon tomato
  purée
1 tablespoon lemon juice
2 spring onions,
  finely chopped

Place the cubes of chicken in a bowl and toss with the Chilli and Garlic sauce and the oil. Leave to marinate for an hour or two.

To make the sauce, mix all ingredients in a small saucepan and heat gently. Meanwhile thread the chicken cubes onto well-soaked wooden satay sticks or steel kebab sticks and grill or barbecue on a medium heat for 10 minutes or until cooked, turning halfway through. Add any marinade left in the bowl to the satay sauce. Serve the satay sticks with the sauce, garnished with salad leaves and spring onions. *Note*: You can freeze the marinated uncooked meat in a bag or container as long as the chicken or pork wasn't previously frozen. Thaw and proceed with cooking as above. The sauce will keep in the fridge for several days and will also freeze.

MEAT

Chilli con Carne

240 calories per portion
Suitable to freeze or will keep in fridge for a day

10 oz/275 g very lean (less than 10% fat) minced beef

1 large onion, finely chopped

1 green pepper, de-seeded and chopped

1 carrot, peeled and finely chopped

1 × 14 oz/400 g can red kidney beans, drained

1 × 14 oz/400 g can chopped tomatoes

1 tablespoon tomato purée

beef stock cube in ¼ pint/140 ml water

1 teaspoon chilli powder (or to taste)

1 tablespoon corn oil

Heat the oil in a non-stick frying pan and sauté the onion until soft and transparent. Add the beef and sauté until browned. Add the rest of the ingredients, stir, cover and simmer for 30 minutes or until vegetables are tender. Taste and add a little salt if liked.

Note: Vegetarians could substitute soya mince for the beef and use a vegetable stock cube.

Liver in Mustard Sauce

265 calories per portion
Not suitable to freeze or store

12 oz/325 g lambs' or calves' liver, sliced very thinly
¼ oz/7 g (1 teaspoon) butter

1 dessertspoon corn oil
1 × 8 oz/225 g pot Greek strained yogurt
3 teaspoons Dijon mustard

Heat the butter and oil in a non-stick frying pan and when it is sizzling but not yet turned brown, add the liver slices and sauté on high for just one minute each side. Remove pan from heat for a minute and remove liver from pan onto a warmed dish. Add the yogurt and mustard to the pan, stir until sauce is hot but not boiling. Add any juices that have by now run off the liver and stir. Serve the sauce poured over the liver.

Note: Use English mustard for a hotter flavour. The sauce is also good with lean steak or a frozen lamb or beef steaklet, and calorie count will remain about the same.

Beef and Pepper Stir-Fry

320 calories per portion
Suitable for freezing or will keep in fridge for a day

1 lb/450 g lean beef steak, cut into bite-sized strips
8 oz/225 g red pepper, de-seeded and cut into strips
4 oz/110 g sweetcorn, frozen
1 dessertspoon corn oil
1 teaspoon Tabasco (hot chilli sauce)

1 tablespoon soya sauce
1 teaspoon honey
1 heaped teaspoon cornflour blended with a little beef stock from cube
approx 200 ml beef stock
4 oz/110 g dried noodles, cooked according to packet instructions

Heat the oil in a wok or non-stick frying pan and add the beef, stirring until it is all browned. Add the pepper and stir a further two minutes, then add the sweetcorn, Tabasco, soya sauce, honey and approx 4 fl oz/100 ml stock and continue stirring for two more minutes. Add the cornflour mixture and noodles and stir to heat through, adding a little more stock if necessary.

Note: You can use fillet of pork in this recipe instead of the beef – or even chicken. The calorie count will remain approximately the same.

Beef Stroganoff

250 calories per portion
Suitable for freezing or will keep in a fridge for a day

16 oz/450 g beef steak, cut into bite-sized strips
10 oz/275 g button mushrooms, sliced
1 Spanish onion, finely chopped
½ oz/15 g butter
1 level tablespoon paprika
2 tablespoons dry sherry
¼ pint/140 ml beef stock from cube
1 heaped teaspoon cornflour blended with a little beef stock
1 × 5 fl oz/140 ml carton soured cream
black pepper and a little salt

Heat the butter in a non-stick frying pan and sauté the onion until transparent. Add the beef, stirring until brown and keeping the heat up high. Add mushrooms and stir for a further minute.

Add paprika and sherry and allow to bubble. Add stock and cornflour mixture and bring to simmer, then take off heat and stir in the soured cream. Check taste and add seasoning if necessary. Before serving sprinkle over some paprika.

Note: You could use braising or stewing steak trimmed of all fat in this recipe for a more economical dish. In that case, after adding the stock, cover and simmer for 1-2 hours, or until meat is tender, before adding cornflour and soured cream.

VEGETARIAN

Vegetable and Lentil Lasagne

340 calories per portion
Not suitable for freezing but will keep in a fridge for up to two days

8 sheets 'no need to
   pre-cook' lasagne
1 × 14 oz/400 g can
   chopped tomatoes
8 oz/225 g courgettes,
   sliced
1 × 8 oz/225 g
   aubergine, cubed
1 large onion, sliced
1 large green pepper,
   de-seeded and sliced
2 oz/50 g green lentils
   (dry weight), boiled
1 tablespoon olive oil

1 teaspoon ground
   coriander
black pepper and a little
   salt
approx 10 fl oz/275 ml
   vegetable stock
For the topping:
2 × 4½ oz/125 g pots
   natural low-fat yogurt
2 medium-sized eggs
3 tablespoons grated
   Parmesan cheese

Heat the oil in a non-stick frying pan and sauté the onion for a few minutes until soft and transparent. Add courgettes and aubergine and stir-fry for a few minutes. Add tomatoes, pepper, lentils, coriander, seasoning and approx 4 fl oz/100 ml of the stock, cover and simmer for 20 minutes or until vegetables are tender (test aubergine with skewer). Add more stock until you have a fairly liquid mixture – if it's too dry the lasagne won't cook properly as the 'no pre-cook' variety soaks up a lot of liquid.

In a suitable ovenproof dish, spread a layer of vegetable mixture followed by half the lasagne sheets, then more vegetable mixture and the remaining four lasagne sheets.

Beat together the eggs and yogurt with a little salt and pepper and spread evenly over the top of the lasagne. Sprinkle the cheese over evenly, and bake at 190°C/375°F/Mark 5 for 40 minutes or until the top is golden.

Note: You can use ordinary lasagne which will need pre-boiling as instructed on packet. In this case there is no need to make the vegetable mixture too runny, so less stock will be needed.

Also note – if you have time, it is wise to salt and drain the aubergine and courgettes as in the following recipe, which will prevent any hint of bitter-ness in these vegetables. However it isn't vital as the longer cooking time seems to diminish any bitter taste and some varieties of courgette are not at all bitter.

Ratatouille Cheese

185 calories per portion
Not suitable for freezing but will keep in a fridge for one to two days

1 × 10oz/275g
  aubergine
10oz/275g courgettes
1 × 6oz/175g green
  pepper, de-seeded
  and sliced
1 × 14oz/400g can
  tomatoes
1 Spanish onion, thinly
  sliced

1 teaspoon basil
1 tablespoon olive oil
black pepper and a little
  salt
6oz/175g reduced-fat
  Cheddar-style cheese,
  grated

Slice the courgettes and aubergine, sprinkle them with salt in a colander set on a plate and allow them to drain for as long as possible. Rinse them and dry in kitchen paper.

Heat the oil in a non-stick frying pan and sauté the onion until soft and transparent. Add the aubergine, courgettes and pepper and sauté for a minute or two. Add the tomatoes, basil and black pepper and simmer, covered, for 20 minutes or until aubergine is tender.

Taste and add salt as necessary. Divide the ratatouille between four gratin dishes, sprinkle over the grated cheese and grill under a medium heat until the cheese is golden.

Note: For a change the Cheddar-style cheese could be omitted. Instead break an egg onto the top of each dish of ratatouille, then sprinkle with a dessert-spoonful of grated Parmesan cheese on each. Bake at 180°C/350°F/Mark 4 for 15 minutes or until eggs are set. Calorie count is the same.

Spicy Bean Casserole

205 calories per portion
Suitable for freezing, although beans may go slightly 'mushy' – will keep in the fridge for a day

1 medium onion, sliced
1 large carrot, sliced
2 sticks celery, chopped
4 oz/110 g sweetcorn, frozen
1 × 14 oz/400 g can red kidney beans, drained and rinsed
1 × 14 oz/400 g can butter beans, drained and rinsed
1 × 14 oz/400 g can tomatoes

1 tablespoon tomato purée
1 teaspoon brown sugar
1 clove garlic, crushed
9 fl oz/275 ml vegetable stock from cube
1 teaspoon chilli powder
1 teaspoon ground cumin seed
salt and black pepper to taste

Pour the tomatoes into a suitable casserole dish and mix in half the vegetable stock, tomato purée and sugar. Add all the remaining ingredients (*except* the rest of the stock), stirring gently. Cover and simmer for approximately 30 minutes, adding extra stock if casserole seems too dry and simmering for few minutes more.

Note: When the celery is tender, the casserole will be ready. You can use different combinations of beans for a change.

Vegetable and Lentil Curry

230 calories per portion
Suitable for freezing and will keep in a fridge for a day or two

4 oz/110 g brown lentils (raw weight)
1 large onion, chopped
1 clove garlic, chopped
1 tablespoon corn oil
8 oz/225 g cauliflower florets
7 oz/200 g potato, cubed, parboiled and drained
1 × 6 oz/175 g aubergine, cubed
4 oz/110 g green beans

1 × 14 oz/400 g can tomatoes
1 tablespoon tomato purée
1 oz/25 g sultanas
1 teaspoon brown sugar
1 tablespoon curry powder of choice (more or less to taste)
5 fl oz/140 ml vegetable stock
1 tablespoon lemon juice

Boil the lentils in 18 fl oz/500 ml water for 30 minutes or until tender. Drain and use some of the water to make the vegetable stock. Heat the oil in a pan and sauté the onion until soft. Add the garlic and curry powder and sauté, stirring, for a minute. Add the remaining ingredients, cover and simmer for 30 minutes or until all vegetables are tender and you have a rich sauce.

Note: Calabrese, carrot or courgettes can be substituted for the cauliflower, aubergine and beans if you like.

Mushroom Risotto

250 calories per portion
Not suitable for freezing but will keep in a fridge for a day

7 oz/200 g risotto or
  patna rice (uncooked)
1 medium onion, finely
  chopped
1 large aubergine
7 oz/200 g mushrooms,
  sliced
1 clove garlic, crushed
1 tablespoon olive oil
1 medium red pepper,
  de-seeded and
  chopped

2 oz/50 g frozen peas
2 tomatoes, skinned,
  de-seeded and
  chopped
1 pint/550 ml vegetable
  stock from cube
black pepper and a little
  salt
1 teaspoon oregano

Chop the aubergine, sprinkle it with salt in a colander and allow to drain for 30 minutes. Rinse and dry in kitchen paper. Heat oil in a large non-stick frying pan and sauté onion until soft and transparent. Add rice and stir to coat. Add garlic and most of stock and bring to simmer.

After 10 minutes add aubergine and continue cooking. When rice is plump and nearly all liquid is absorbed add rest of ingredients and cook for further few minutes, adding a little more stock if required.
Note: Brown rice can also be used for this dish. Allow an extra 15 minutes cooking time.

SALADS

Spanish Salad

285 calories per portion
Not suitable for freezing but will keep in a fridge for a day maximum

11½oz/325g cooked peeled prawns
4½oz/125g brown rice (uncooked)
4 spring onions, chopped
1 medium ripe avocado
1 small green and 1 small red pepper, de-seeded and chopped

4oz/110g cucumber, chopped
4floz/110ml oil-free French dressing

Boil the rice with a little salt in 12 fl oz/325 ml water with a level teaspoon of turmeric added, until rice is tender. Drain, and when cooled add the onions, peppers, prawns and cucumber. Peel the avocado, slice it and add immediately to the salad with the dressing to prevent it turning brown. Toss salad gently and serve on bed of lettuce.

Note: You can also use white long grain rice in this recipe, in which case you could add a pinch of saffron to the rice water for an added touch of luxury, instead of the turmeric.

Egg and Tuna Salad

190 calories per portion
Not suitable for freezing but will keep in a fridge for a day

14 oz/400 g tuna in
  brine, drained
4 medium-sized eggs
  hard-boiled,
  quartered
4 tomatoes, not too ripe,
  quartered
4 oz/100 g cucumber,
  chopped

1 bunch watercress,
  washed and chopped,
  leaving a few sprigs
  whole
4 tablespoons oil-free
  French dressing
lettuce leaves

In a bowl, gently combine all the ingredients except the lettuce. Arrange lettuce leaves on the serving plates and divide salad between them, garnishing with extra watercress leaves.

Spiced Chicken in Tomatoes

150 calories per portion
Not suitable for freezing but will keep in a fridge for a day

4 beef tomatoes (approx
  4 1/2 oz/140 g each)
4 oz/110 g cooked brown
  rice (cooked weight)
6 oz/175 g cooked lean
  chicken meat, diced
  fairly small
1 oz/25 g sultanas
4 spring onions, chopped
2 sticks tender celery,
  chopped small
3 tablespoons natural
  low-fat yogurt

1 1/2 tablespoons
  reduced-calorie
  mayonnaise
1 level teaspoon mild
  curry powder
1 good teaspoon tomato
  purée
1 teaspoon lemon juice
black pepper and a little
  salt

Cut the top quarter off each tomato (stalk end) and scoop out the seeds and pulp. Combine the yogurt, seasoning, mayonnaise, curry powder, lemon juice and tomato purée in a bowl then add the rice, chicken, sultanas, onions, and celery and toss all together well. Fill the tomatoes with the mixture.

Garnish with chopped parsley if liked.

Note: Turkey meat or cooked smoked cod, flaked, works well in this dish instead of the chicken. Calorie count would be the same for the turkey, and 125 calories per portion for the cod.

Tabbouleh

195 calories per portion
Not suitable for freezing but will keep for up to two days in a fridge

4 oz/110 g bulgar
   (pre-cooked cracked
   wheat)
2 tomatoes, peeled and
   chopped
2 spring onions, chopped
1 bunch parsley,
   chopped
4 oz/110 g cucumber,
   chopped

1 bunch mint, chopped
1 1/4 tablespoons olive oil
1 tablespoon lemon juice
2 medium-sized eggs,
   hard-boiled
black pepper and a little
   salt

Steep the bulgar in 6 fl oz/175 ml boiling water and let stand for 10 minutes. Drain and allow to dry on kitchen paper, then transfer it to a serving bowl. Combine with all the remaining ingredients except the egg. Quarter the eggs and arrange them on top of the dish, garnishing with a few sprigs of parsley.
Note: Parsley, mint and other herbs can be frozen in yogurt pots during the summer so that you always

have some available through the winter — dried parsley and mint is not suitable.

Pasta and Tuna Salad

195 calories per portion
Not suitable for freezing but will keep in a fridge for a day or two

7 oz/200 g tuna in brine, drained

12 oz/325 g cooked wholewheat pasta shapes of choice

1 medium green pepper, de-seeded and chopped

8 spring onions, chopped

1 red dessert apple

handful fresh parsley, chopped

1 × 5 fl oz/140 ml tub natural low-fat yogurt

2 tablespoons reduced-calorie mayonnaise

1 teaspoon tomato purée

pinch chilli powder

1 teaspoon lemon juice

black pepper and a little salt

Combine the pasta, pepper, onions, half the parsley and tuna in a serving bowl. Combine the yogurt, mayonnaise, tomato purée, chilli, lemon juice and seasoning. Core and chop the apple and add to the salad. Pour over the dressing, stir gently. Garnish with remaining parsley.

Chicken and Walnut Pasta Salad

300 calories per portion
Not suitable for freezing but will keep in a fridge for a day

10 oz/275 g cooked
   chicken meat, diced
12 oz/325 g cooked
   wholewheat pasta
   shapes of choice
1 red dessert apple
1½ oz/40 g shelled
   walnut pieces
4 sticks tender celery,
   chopped

1 × 5 fl oz/140 ml tub
   natural low-fat yogurt
2 tablespoons
   reduced-calorie
   mayonnaise
1 tablespoon lemon juice
black pepper and a little
   salt
a little parsley, chopped

Combine the yogurt, mayonnaise, lemon juice and seasoning. Combine the chicken, pasta, walnut and celery in a serving dish. Core and chop the apple at the last minute and add it with the dressing. Toss and serve garnished with chopped parsley.

Peanut Coleslaw

185 calories per portion
Not suitable for freezing but will keep in a fridge for two days

12 oz/325 g carrot,
   grated

1 × 5 fl oz/140 ml tub
   natural low-fat yogurt

12 oz/325 g white
cabbage, shredded
1 small onion, finely
chopped
2 oz/50 g fresh shelled
unsalted peanuts

1 1/2 fl oz/40 ml
unsweetened orange
juice
2 oz/50 g raisins
black pepper and a little
salt

Combine all the ingredients in a bowl and serve.

Pasta Salad with Chilli Dressing

285 calories per portion
Not suitable for freezing but will keep for two days
in a fridge

1 lb/450 g cooked weight
pasta shells
2 large green peppers,
de-seeded and
chopped
8 spring onions, chopped
8 black olives, stoned,
chopped
6 oz/175 g feta cheese,
crumbled
small bunch parsley,
chopped
Dressing:
4 oz/110 ml oil-free
French dressing

2 level tablespoons
tomato purée
2 level tablespoons
water
3 oz/75 g cucumber,
peeled and finely
chopped
1 teaspoon dried basil *or*
8 fresh basil
leaves, chopped
1 tablespoon Chilli &
Garlic sauce (e.g.
Lea & Perrins)
2 teaspoons brown
sugar

Combine all the dressing ingredients well – a whizz in a blender will give a smoother sauce. Combine all the salad ingredients in the serving bowl, pour the dressing over and toss lightly.

Rice and Smoked Fish Salad

210 calories per portion
Not suitable for freezing but will keep in a fridge for a day

1 lb/450 g smoked cod
   or haddock fillet,
   skinned and flaked
12 oz/325 g cooked
   weight brown rice
1 bunch watercress,
   washed and chopped
1 small bunch parsley,
   chopped
8 oz/225 g button
   mushrooms, sliced

1 small red pepper,
   de-seeded and
   chopped
Dressing:
4½ oz/125 ml oil-free
   French dressing
1 good teaspoon Dijon
   mustard
pinch brown sugar

Combine all dry ingredients in serving bowl, taking care not to break down the fish too much, then pour over the dressing combined with the mustard and sugar and toss very lightly.

Note: Other smoked fish, such as smoked trout, smoked mackerel (or even smoked salmon!) are much higher in calories than smoked cod and haddock and they should not be used in this recipe.

SAUCES, DIPS AND SOUP

Hot Bolognese Mushroom Sauce

175 calories per portion
Suitable for freezing or will keep in a fridge for a day

10 oz/275 g very lean (less than 10% fat) minced beef
8 oz/225 g mushrooms, sliced
1 medium onion, finely chopped
1 carrot, finely chopped
1 × 14 oz/400 g can tomatoes, chopped
2 tablespoons tomato purée
1 clove garlic, crushed
1 fl oz/25 ml red wine
1 teaspoon Tabasco
little beef stock from cube
salt and black pepper
1 dessertspoon olive oil

Heat the oil in a non-stick frying pan and sauté the onion until it is soft and transparent. Add the garlic and beef and cook, stirring, until the beef is browned. Add the wine and allow to bubble. Add the carrot, tomatoes, mushrooms and tomato purée. Tabasco and seasoning and bring to simmer. Add a little beef stock, cover and simmer for 30 minutes, adding extra beef stock if mixture looks too dry.
Note: This sauce is good with baked potatoes and in lasagne as well as with spaghetti.

Hot Barbecue Sauce

42 calories per portion
Suitable for freezing or will keep for several days in a fridge
Suitable for vegetarians

1 tablespoon olive oil
2 tablespoons tomato
   purée
½ teaspoon garlic purée
   or 1 clove garlic, well
   crushed
1 tablespoon red wine
   vinegar
1 teaspoon Dijon
   mustard

1 teaspoon honey
1 teaspoon
   Worcestershire sauce
1 level teaspoon ground
   chilli

Heat the oil in a small saucepan then add the remaining ingredients, stirring. Simmer for a minute.
Note: Made as above, this is a good coating sauce for all types of barbecued, grilled or baked meat or fish. Mixed with a little water it could also be served as a side sauce.

Tomato Sauce

70 calories per portion
Suitable for freezing or will keep in a fridge for a day

1 tablespoon olive oil   2 fl oz/50 ml white wine

1 Spanish onion, finely
  chopped
1 × 14oz/400g can
  chopped tomatoes
1 teaspoon
  Worcestershire sauce
1 clove garlic, crushed

1 teaspoon brown sugar
1 tablespoon tomato
  purée
1 teaspoon chopped
  basil
salt and black pepper to
  taste

Heat the oil in a saucepan and add the onion, stirring for a few minutes until soft. Add the wine and allow to bubble. Add the rest of the ingredients, stir and simmer for 15 minutes or until you have a rich sauce. For a smoother sauce, purée in a blender.

Note: For variety, try adding 8oz/225g sliced mushrooms to the sauce, stirring them in to the onions before adding rest of the ingredients. This will add 8 calories a portion.

Spicy Cheese Dip

115 calories per portion
Suitable for freezing if re-beaten after thawing, or will keep in a fridge for two or three days

11½oz/325g skimmed
  milk soft cheese *or*
  drained tofu
2fl oz/50ml skimmed
  milk

1 small clove garlic,
  crushed
1 teaspoon Tabasco
1 dessertspoon lemon
  juice

3 tablespoons
reduced-calorie
mayonnaise
small bunch watercress,
washed and finely
chopped

salt and black pepper to
taste

Blend all ingredients in blender or by hand.
Note: For a change, omit the watercress and instead
add either 1 teaspoon curry powder or 2 teaspoons
tomato purée.

Lentil Dip

140 calories per portion
Suitable for freezing or will keep in a fridge for two or
three days

3½oz/100g (dry
weight)
brown lentils
1 tablespoon olive oil
1 × 5floz/140ml tub
natural low-fat yogurt
1 tablespoon lemon juice
½ teaspoon ground
cumin

1 tablespoon chopped
parsley plus parsley to
garnish
black pepper and a little
salt

Cook the lentils in boiling water for about 30 minutes
or until tender. Drain them and put them in a blender

with the rest of the ingredients and blend until just smooth. Serve garnished with parsley.
Note: For a coarser dip, blend the ingredients by hand.

Gazpacho Soup

100 calories per portion
Suitable for freezing (excluding garnishes) or will keep in a fridge for two days

1 × 12 oz/325 g
   cucumber, peeled and
   chopped
2 × 14 oz/400 g cans
   chopped tomatoes
1 green pepper,
   de-seeded and
   chopped
1 Spanish onion,
   chopped
1 large clove garlic,
   crushed
1 tablespoon wine
   vinegar

1 tablespoon olive oil
1 teaspoon chilli powder
black pepper and salt to
   taste
Garnishes:
1 slice wholemeal bread,
   toasted and cubed
chopped cucumber,
   tomato, pepper, spring
   onions
chopped parsley

Blend all the ingredients, except the garnishes, in a blender. Add a little water if soup seems too thick and re-blend. Serve topped with the garnishes (included in calorie count).

CHAPTER SIX

The High Speed Slimming Exercise Programme

I recently read a report from the British Heart Foundation that said that while 83% of UK adults say they would like to take some regular exercise, only 40% of males and 25% of females actually do anything regular at all, including walking. So should you by any chance be one of the remaining percentage of men and women who prefer to *think* about exercise rather than actually *doing* it, I will suggest that you return now to Chapter Three and re-read all the amazing benefits that a little regular exercise can work on your body – and, most importantly, on your slimming campaign.

The benefits are worth repeating in shortened form here so that they are etched on your memory every day and especially for whenever the urge to shirk the programme in this chapter becomes strong:

• Exercise burns up many calories while you are actually doing it – many, many more than just sitting around will do.
• Aerobic exercise increases your metabolic rate for up to 24 hours *after* you have done it.

- Exercise burns off *fat* but puts on *lean tissue*. Lean tissue is much more metabolically active than fat tissue and so here's another way exercise is helping you burn up calories. Also, lean tissue gives you a fit, shapely, lean look rather than the slim but unshapely look many dieters get who do NO exercise.
- Exercise can lose you inches where you want them to go – something that dieting alone cannot achieve.
- Exercise prevents the 'sag effect' that many slimmers – particularly ones who are a great deal overweight – experience.
- If you exercise, you can eat *more* but lose weight *faster*.

Right, so, filled with enthusiasm at the reminder of all the benefits of exercise, why not make a start now?

The *High Speed Slimming* exercise programme consists of *two* routines that I would like you to do almost every day. There is an *AM* PLAN – a programme of stretching, toning and strength exercises that you should do in the morning, preferably after your breakfast. This will take you around 20 minutes, and I have designed it to maximize *lean tissue build* and to *reshape* you speedily.

Then there is a *PM* PLAN – an aerobic programme to allow you to burn up hundreds of extra calories and to increase your metabolic rate permanently. The *PM* PLAN will also, incidentally, increase your lean tissue and, depending on which aerobic activity you choose, help to reshape you too. The *PM* PLAN is also 20 minutes a day, and should be done in the early evening, preferably after your tea.

I have designed the exercise programme in two separate parts for two main reasons. Firstly, for your convenience. I find it much easier to fit two short sessions of exercise into my day rather than one long one and so I believe you will too. And you are much more likely to stick with something that is convenient than with something that isn't. You do the *AM* PLAN in your own bedroom or sitting room. The activity choices in the *PM* PLAN are mostly ones you will do outdoors or in a place other than your home.

Secondly, you get more metabolic benefit from spacing your exercise out like this than you would if you did it all in one session. The morning session will increase the oxygen in your system and help you to burn up the calories in what you eat all day. The evening session will ensure that what you eat from afternoon onwards will be used as fuel rather than stored on your body as fat.

For some people it may be more convenient to do the aerobic *PM* PLAN in the morning and the toning *AM* PLAN later in the day. In that case you can swop the programmes around – but remember, never crawl out of bed and straight into an aerobic routine. You must allow some time for your body to warm up and for your heart to get going, which is why I would prefer it if you can do the aerobic plan as suggested here.

You should do the plans six days a week throughout your slimming campaign. Once you reach your target weight and shape, do each plan at least three times a week — not necessarily on the same day. You could do the *AM* PLAN every other morning and the *PM* PLAN on alternate evenings, for instance.

THE *AM* PLAN

This plan consists of:

* a WARM-UP
* two STRETCHING exercises
* eight STRENGTH AND TONE exercises, many of which have an *easy* and a *harder* version
* three more STRETCHES which also act as the cool down

The whole routine should take you 20 minutes — though for the first day or two you'll need to spend a little longer getting acclimatized to the routine. Before you begin, read these notes carefully:

* Do the routine before noon every day — but don't get straight out of bed and go directly into the routine. At the very minimum, take a warm bath first. Your limbs may be a little stiff and unyielding if you do the routine on waking.

• Exercise in a warm room, preferably in a stretch bodysuit or leotard, but shorts and a T-shirt will do. There are no high-impact exercises in the routine so you needn't wear training shoes, but I find a soft pair of leather jazz shoes comfortable.

• Exercises 3 to 10 have an *easier* version (shown in the main photo) and a *harder* version (shown in the small photo). Everyone should start on the easier versions of these exercises then, when they can do them well, progress to the harder versions.

Most of the harder versions involve the use of dumb-bells or wrist weights and/or ankle weights. A set of ankle and wrist weights is not too expensive. If you prefer you can use heavy food cans, such as baked bean tins, or bottles of cooking oil, instead of dumb-bells, although they are slightly more awkward to hold than dumb-bells.

Doing the harder versions of the exercises will simply mean quicker toning and a greater degree of strengthening – in other words, you'll build more lean body tissue (muscle) than if you just stay with the easier exercises. The harder exercises will help you to slim faster!

Warm-up

1. Stand, relaxed, and spend half a minute breathing steadily and deeply (Figure 1) – feel your ribcage expand and contract.

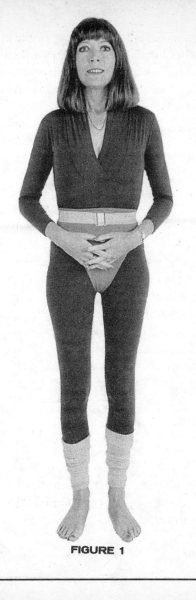

FIGURE 1

2. Now spend half a minute doing small, quick steps on the spot, flexing ankles in a rhythmic movement, carrying weight on balls of feet (Figure 2). At the same time, shake hands loosely at sides. Smile!

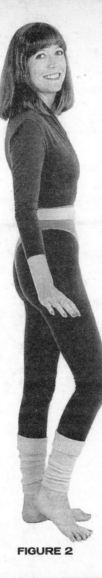

FIGURE 2

3. Do half a minute high step marching (Figure 3) – lifting knees high off floor, breathing deeply and steadily, and swinging arms widely back and forward as if really marching.

4. Lastly, using a very sturdy wooden box or stool, about 12″ high, or a stair if there is one handy, do one minute of stepping (Figure 4). This means you stand directly in front of the step or box and step up on to it, first with one foot leading, then with the other, i.e. left foot up, right foot up, left foot down, right foot down, then right foot up, left foot up, right foot down, left foot down. That sequence counts as two steps – do 30 steps in all, which should take you about a minute.

That ends the warm-up and by now your heart rate should be slightly increased, you should feel warm and relaxed. Now it's on to two stretching exercises.

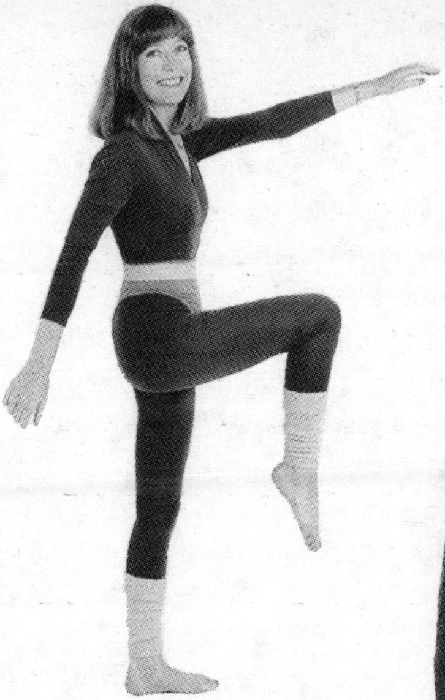

FIGURE 3

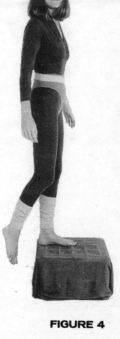

FIGURE 4

Exercise one

A stretch to define and slim your waistline which will also help to stretch out your ribcage and loosen shoulders. It consists of two movements. First, stand, legs together, preferably back against a wall. Place right hand on hip then reach up to the ceiling with your left hand, keeping back and hips straight (Figure 5). If you have poor shoulder mobility, your left hand may not be able to touch the wall behind you – you will soon improve. Reach as far towards the ceiling as you can; feel the stretch along your left side and hold this for 15 seconds. Repeat with right arm.

Now place right hand just above right knee, which should be slightly bent, reach over towards your right side with your left arm as shown (Figure 6). The effectiveness of this exercise is minimized if you don't keep your spine aligned with the wall. Feel the stretch along your left side, hold for 15 seconds. Repeat to the other side.

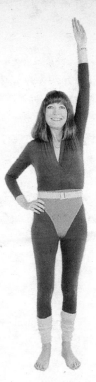

FIGURE 5

FIGURE 6

Exercise two

A stretch to release tight hamstrings (the muscles at the back and sides of your leg which are very tight in many people) and to help mobilize your hips. It will also improve the shape and tone of your hips and thighs.

Sit on a towel on the floor, left leg bent at knee as shown, so that your heel comes as far in towards your groin as it can without strain. Extend your right leg as shown keeping upper body slightly forward and supporting yourself on your hands in front of your body (Figure 7). Feel the stretch all along the straight leg. Hold for a count of 30 seconds, then repeat to the other side.

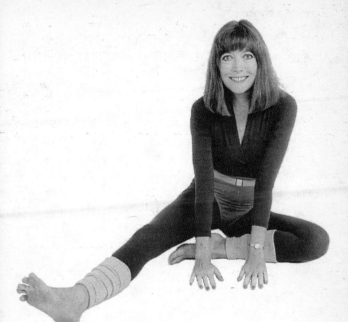

FIGURE 7

Exercise three

These relatively easy push-ups will build strength in your arms and chest and help to eliminate upper-arm flab.

Easier: Kneel on all fours as shown, fingers pointing inwards and arms directly under chest (Figure 8). Now slowly lower your upper body towards the floor as far as you can go and slowly return to a count of six for the complete movement (Figure 9). Repeat 10 times. (You may not be able to manage 10 at first, but build up to 10 as quickly as you can).

Harder: Move your knees back so that more weight is on your upper body and do the push-ups as before (Figure 10).

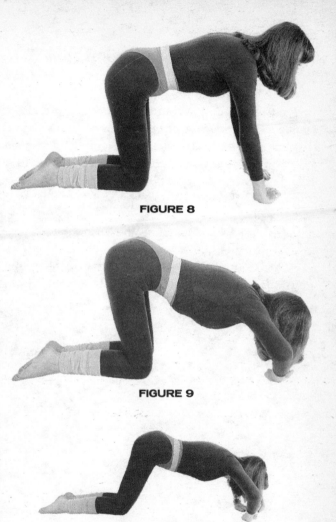

FIGURE 8

FIGURE 9

FIGURE 10

Exercise four

This curl-back movement is for stomach strength and tone. It is important to do the exercise slowly and to feel the pull in your stomach only.

Easier: Sit on towel with knees bent and feet flat on floor as shown. Keeping back straight and stomach pulled in, raise arms parallel to floor (Figure 11). Now very slowly curl back your upper body to a 45° angle and hold this position, breathing easily, for a count of 10 (Figure 12). Slowly return to start and repeat 5 times.

Harder: Slowly continue the curl until you are lying back on the floor – you must do this as slowly as possible (Figure 13). Using your arms to help you, return to start position and repeat 5 times.

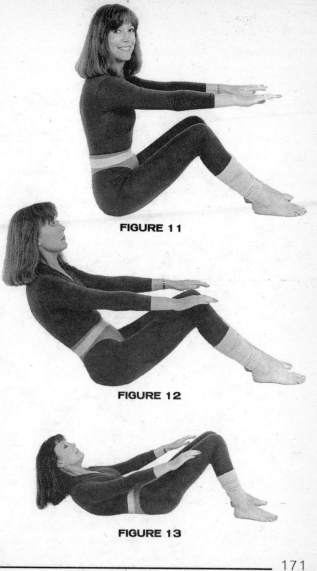

FIGURE 11

FIGURE 12

FIGURE 13

Exercise five

These pelvic lifts are wonderful for lifting and tightening a saggy bottom and also help to work the thighs and stomach muscles a little, too.

Easier: Lie on back on towel, arms crossed over chest, knees bent (Figure 14). Now, using your bottom muscles, pull your lower body about 3″, off the floor, hold for a count of 6 seconds then return to floor and repeat 10 times (Figure 15). While you are holding, really try to squeeze your bottom together hard.

Harder: Once you have reached the 'hold' position, extend your right leg straight out in front of you (Figure 16). You will find that your left bottom is working harder now. Alternate legs with each of the ten repeats.

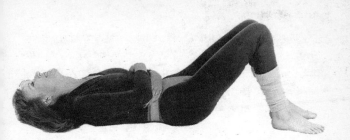

FIGURE 14

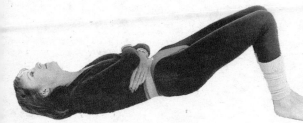

FIGURE 15

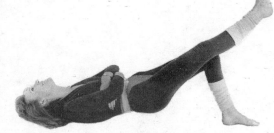

FIGURE 16

Exercise six

Side leg lifts will quickly strengthen and tone your outer thighs and will also work your hips and bottom.

Easier: Lie on your right side on a towel, upper body weight supported on elbow, left hand out in front of you and right leg slightly bent (Figure 17). Now raise your left leg as high as it will go until you feel a pull along the inner thigh (Figure 18). Hold for a count of 6 seconds, slowly lower and repeat 10 times. Turn over and repeat on the other side.

Harder: Wear ankle weights to do the exercise as above (Figure 19).

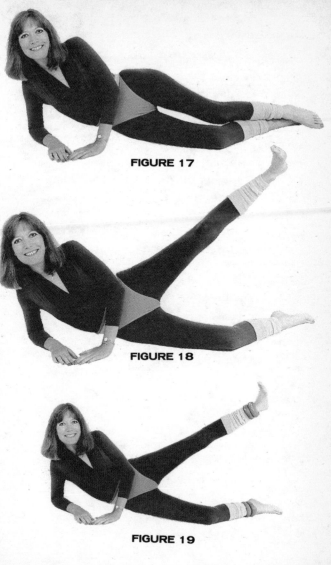

FIGURE 17

FIGURE 18

FIGURE 19

Exercise seven

This kneeling leg lift is great for bottom, hamstrings and lower back strength.

Easier: Kneel on a towel on the floor on elbows, keeping head, neck and back aligned (Figure 20). Now lift right leg out straight behind you until it is also in line with head, neck and back (Figure 21). Feel the pull in your bottom and along top of leg. Hold this position for a count of 15 seconds, lower and repeat to the other side, then repeat both sides again for another count of 15.

Harder: Wear ankle weights to do the exercise as above (Figure 22).

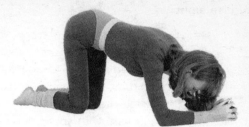

FIGURE 20

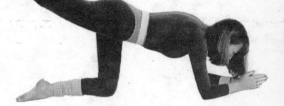

FIGURE 21

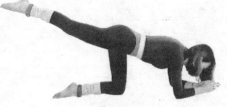

FIGURE 22

Exercise eight

This series of arm exercises is brilliant at shaping arms and building lean tissue. It is also marvellous for strengthening weak shoulders and upper back and for firming the chest/bustline.

Easier: Stand, legs together, as shown (Figure 23). Make two loose fists with your hands and, with palms facing towards chest, pump each arm in turn up towards the ceiling, bringing the arm back down to waist level each time. Count 30 arm pumps altogether.

Now bring arms out to your sides and up until they are parallel to floor (Figure 24). First with palms facing to the back, move arms a few inches backwards, feeling the pull in your shoulders. Move arms back and forward these few inches 10 times, then turn palms round to face front and repeat a further 10 times (Figure 25).

Lastly, bring arms out to the sides and then slowly raise and lower up to 45° above the horizontal, then lower them to 45° below the horizontal, 20 times, as slowly as you can (Figure 26).

Harder: Do each of the movements as above using wrist weights or dumb-bells (Figure 27). If using dumb-bells, start with 1 kg bells. You can progress to heavier weights in time.

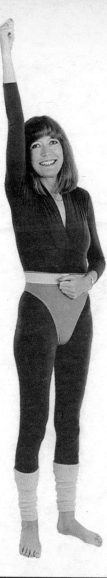

FIGURE 23

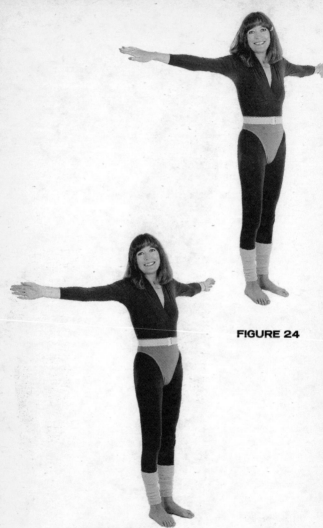

FIGURE 24

FIGURE 25

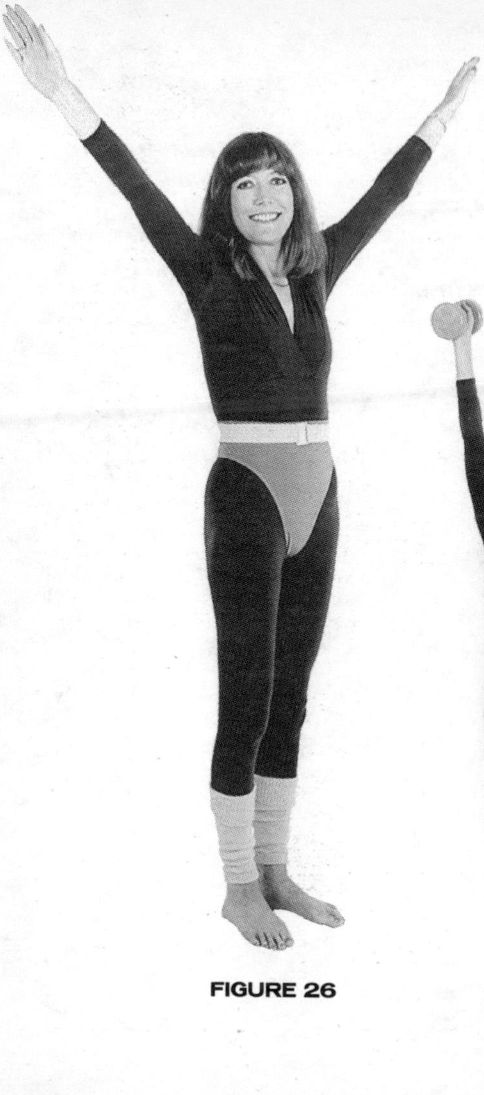

FIGURE 26

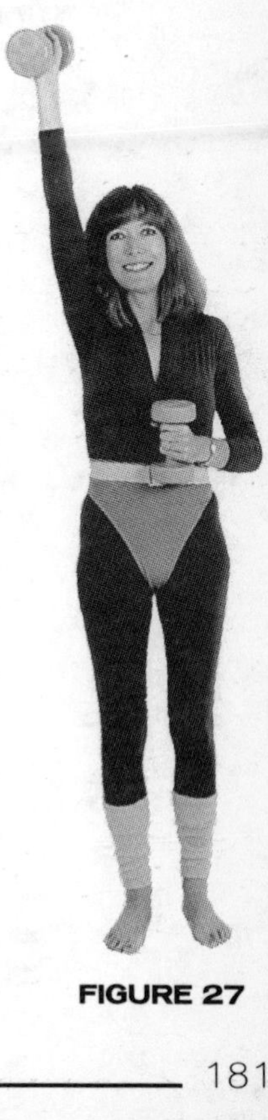

FIGURE 27

Exercise nine

The legs contain the largest muscles in your body so it is important when building lean tissue to do as much work on them as you can. This exercise works the legs, arms and heart at the same time.

Easier: Start from a standing position. Now simply bring your left heel up behind your right leg and at the same time bring your right hand down to meet it, while bringing your left arm up above your head (Figure 28). In a rhythmic sequence, repeat the movement to the other side (Figure 29). Repeat 60 times (each side counts as one repeat).

Harder: Wear ankle and wrist weights to do the exercise as above (Figure 30).

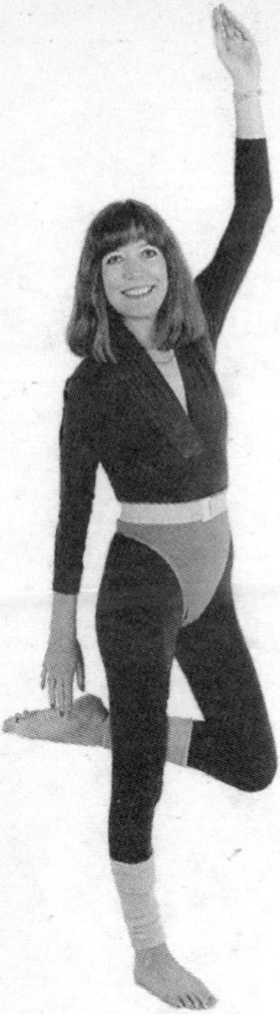

FIGURE 28

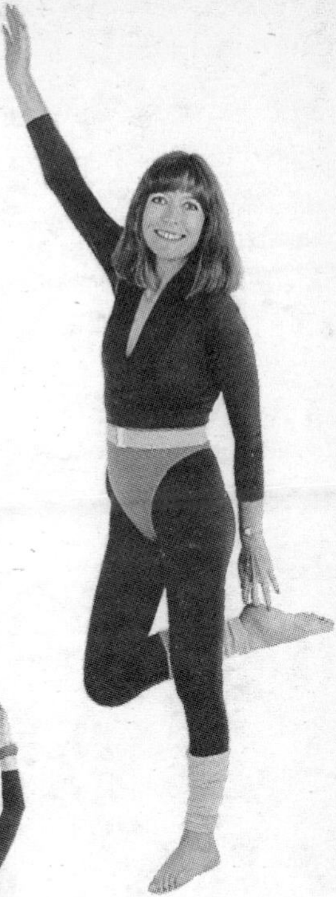

FIGURE 29

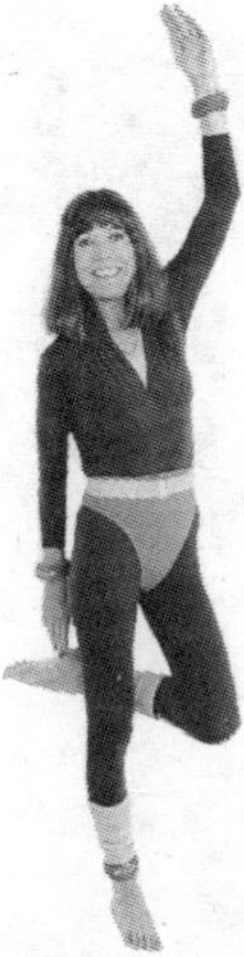

FIGURE 30

Exercise ten

Another great exercise for legs, arms and heart. The secret is to get a good rhythm going.

Easier: Sit on towel, upper body weight resting on arms, knees bent (Figure 31). Lift bottom slightly off floor and now kick out first your left leg then your right (Figure 32). As you do each kick, bend your elbows and lower body towards floor, raising it again to starting position as each leg returns to start. Do 60 of these kicks, i.e. 30 each side.

Harder: Use ankle weights and do the exercise as above (Figure 33).

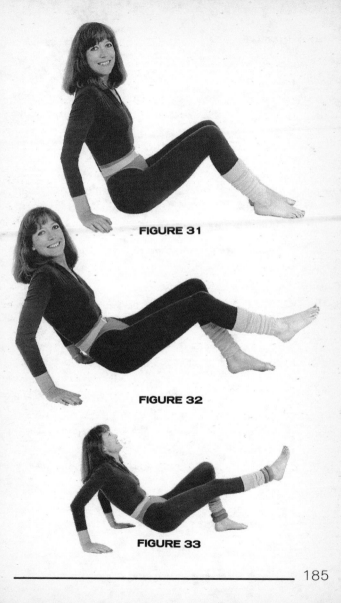

FIGURE 31

FIGURE 32

FIGURE 33

Cool down

The cool down consists of three simple stretches that will relax the parts of your body which have been working hard, as well as cooling you down. The last stretch will also help to tone your body from top to toe.

1.   Lie on towel, knees bent. Bring your right leg in towards your body and clasp behind thigh and calf as shown (Figure 34). Gently pull leg in towards head until you feel a pleasant stretch. Hold for a count of 15 seconds. Repeat to other side.

2.   Now kneel on a towel and curl your body up until bottom is resting on heels, forehead is touching floor and hands are stretched out as far in front of you as they will go (Figure 35). Feel your spine and shoulders stretch out. Hold for a count of 30 seconds.

3.   Turn over and lie on back on floor. Point your toes to the ceiling, push your stomach down into the floor to flatten your lower back, stretch your waist area out by pulling your legs down towards the wall nearest your feet. Put your hands on your stomach and make sure shoulders are flat on the floor (Figure 36). You should now be feeling a stretch all along your upper body and hips. Hold this position for a count of 30 seconds.

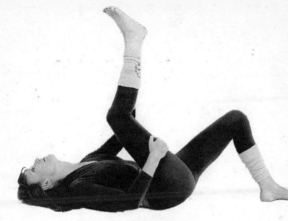

FIGURE 34

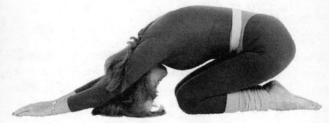

FIGURE 35

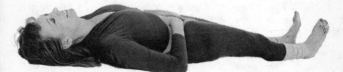

FIGURE 36

Now slowly move arms up and over head until backs of hands are touching floor above head and arms are as close to the floor as you can get them (Figure 37) – all the while maintaining your position as described above. Hold for a count of 30 seconds.

Lastly, bring arms out to sides, concentrating on keeping shoulders flat and backs of hands on floor (Figure 38). Hold this position for a count of 30.

Get up from this final stretch slowly by rolling on to right side and using right arm to push yourself up (Figure 39).

And that's the end of the *AM* PLAN.

THE *PM* PLAN

The *PM* PLAN involves aerobic activity designed to suit *everyone*. It isn't a 'kill or cure' plan that requires you to do anything other than increase the fitness of your heart and lungs in a gradual and sensible way. There is no need to do otherwise – in fact, over-exerting yourself is counterproductive.

Because so many of us do so *little* aerobic activity and are therefore *so* unfit, the British Heart Foundation report that 'brisk walking is sufficiently vigorous ... for more than two-thirds of the population'.

All you do is choose your activity (or activities) from the suggestions described later, and follow the

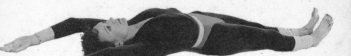

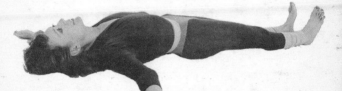

FIGURE 37

FIGURE 38

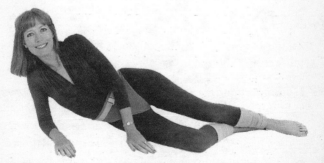

FIGURE 39

three-stage programme designed for each.

But first, a few general guidelines.

Personal preference

If you haven't exercised for years, think back to what you used to enjoy most as a child — or whenever you last did do exercise. There is little point picking something *now* that you didn't like then. For example, if you hated swimming there is little point in picking that as your chosen activity — even if you live next door to a swimming pool — as you are likely to enjoy it even less now. Whatever you choose, you are going to do it for six days a week, minimum 20 minutes a day — so *do pick something you think you will enjoy.*

Convenience

Then again, there is no point picking something you like if it is inconvenient for your situation. If you fancy swimming but the nearest pool is a 45-minute journey away, be honest — you won't stick with the programme, will you? Similarly, there is no point in choosing the cycling programme if you live on the busiest, most dangerous road in town and haven't cycled for 30 years. Choose something you really will be able to fit into your life.

Understanding

In order to get the most out of the *PM* PLAN, you should understand what the programme is going to do for you. You will be gradually increasing your body's need for oxygen by asking your heart and major muscle groups to do more work. They can't work without oxygen and so that is the meaning of the word 'aerobic' – 'with air'. To take in enough air to keep your muscles going while they work, your heart needs to work more efficiently and so do your lungs. Your lungs take in the air and then your heart pumps it round your body in the blood.

If you exercise daily, gradually your heart and lungs will become more and more efficient and so eventually you will need to make your exercise programme *harder* – by increasing resistance or speed in your programme.

If you don't make your programme progressive, soon it won't be aerobic any longer because your heart and lungs will be fitter and easily able to cope with what you are asking of them. So whichever programme you choose, follow the three-stage plan. Most people with moderate to poor levels of fitness (but in reasonable health) will reach Stage Three in four weeks or so, but go at your own pace.

The activities that form the core of the *PM* PLAN are walking (maybe incorporating some jogging), swimming, cycling, exercise cycling, rowing machine, and a combined step/skip/rebound plan. The programmes and notes for each start below. Here are some ways you can vary the *PM* PLAN:

• From time to time (say, once a week) you could exchange one normal *PM* programme for *either* an aerobics class *or* a session of active disco dancing *or* a roller skating session.

• You can mix up to two activities and do each three times a week on alternate days – e.g. walking and swimming, or walking and cycling.

• You can do 1 month on one activity then move on to another one, and so on.

THE WALKING PROGRAMME

Note: This is the preferred choice for many people as it involves no equipment, can be done almost anywhere and can get you from A to B! The British Heart Foundation's definition of 'brisk walking' is 4 mph but in practice it is the pace that gets your heart beating faster and has you slightly breathless, but not so 'out of puff' that you feel uncomfortable/ want to stop/can't talk while walking. Use those criteria then to decide whether or not you are walking 'briskly'.

Wear suitable shoes – cushioned trainers are better than anything else – and if you walk alone, especially after dark, be sensible about where you walk. If you're female I suggest you walk before dark or pick a different activity in the winter months.

If you work within walking distance of home, you may feel inclined to start walking home from work as your daily *PM* PLAN exercise – this may work, but you may find as you get fitter that you need to vary the route home, finding longer alternatives, as what took you 20 minutes in Stage One may take you only 10 or so in Stage Three.

If walking from home, remember that 10 minutes out equals 10 minutes back, so don't walk for 20 minutes in one direction!

Stage One
- Walk on the flat.
- First 5 minutes – slow walking to warm up.
- Second 5 minutes – walk as briskly as you can, obeying the instructions on page 192.
- Third 5 minutes – walk steadily.
- Next 3 minutes – walk as briskly as you can again.
- Last 2 minutes – walk steadily to home.

Stage Two
- First 3 minutes – walk slowly to warm up.
- Next 10 minutes – walk as briskly as you can, obeying the instructions above.
- Next 5 minutes – walk steadily.
- Last 2 minutes – walk slowly to home.

Stage Three
- First 2 minutes – walk steadily to warm up.
- Next 16 minutes – walk as briskly as you can, obeying the instructions above.
- Last 2 minutes – walk steadily to home.

When you have completed Stage Three and find that however fast you walk on the flat you are still breathing normally and your heart rate isn't increased, you can add further progression by walking uphill, by wearing ankle weights or by doing a slow jog instead of the brisk walking.

However, always start and finish the session steadily.

THE CYCLING PROGRAMME

Note: Ideal cycling country contains plenty of flat so that you can build up fitness, but also contains some hills so that you can work harder later. The same rules apply to cycling as to walking — be sensible about cycling alone in remote areas and alone after dark, and 'fast cycling' means the pace that gets you slightly breathless and gets your heart beating faster, but doesn't cause you pain, burning in your legs, or breathlessness to the point where you have to stop and recover.

Wear comfortable clothes and plan out some routes that you can cover in 20 minutes or so.

If you haven't used your bike for years, check it over for safety — brakes, nuts and bolts, punctures, etc.

Stage One
• Cycle on the flat.
• First 5 minutes — slow cycling to warm up.
• Second 5 minutes — fast cycling to achieve exertion as described above.

- Third 5 minutes – steady cycling.
- Next 3 minutes – fast cycling as before.
- Last 2 minutes - slow cycling to home.

Stage Two
- First 3 minutes – steady cycling.
- Next 14 minutes – fast cycling to achieve exertion as described above.
- Last 3 minutes – steady cycling to home.

Stage Three
- First 2 minutes – steady cycling.
- Next 10 minutes – fast cycling as above.
- Next 4 minutes – uphill cycling in same gear (don't stand on pedals).
- Next 2 minutes – cycle downhill.
- Last 2 minutes – steady cycling to home.

When you have completed Stage Three and need to increase the workload, add more hill cycling (but don't count the time spent coasting downhill as part of the 20 minutes) *or* add weights to yourself.

THE SWIMMING PROGRAMME

Note: Swimming is probably the perfect choice if you are very overweight, as exercising in the water means you place little strain on the joints. But bear in mind, even if you have a pool near you, that the 20 minutes' exercise means continuous swimming, which can sometimes be difficult in a crowded pool. So try to go at a time when the pool isn't so busy.

Lengths that follow are for a 25-metre pool.

Stage One

- First 2 minutes – warm up by standing up to shoulder level in water and practising breast-stroke and crawl arm strokes, 1 minute, then hold edge of bath and practise leg strokes for breast-stroke and crawl.
- Now do 2 lengths' breast-stroke steadily, pause for 20 seconds then do 2 lengths' crawl.
- Repeat this for another 10 minutes, then finish with 2 minutes back-stroke.

Stage Two

- First 5 minutes – 5 lengths' breast-stroke.
- Next 5 minutes – 8 lengths' crawl.
- Next 5 minutes – 5 lengths' breast-stroke.
- Next 3 minutes – 5 lengths' crawl.
- Last 2 minutes – 2 lengths' back-stroke.

Stage Three

- First 2 minutes – 2 lengths' breast-stroke.
- Next 16 minutes – as many lengths' crawl as you can do. If you get overtired, revert to breast-stroke for 1 length.
- Last 2 minutes – 2 lengths' back-stroke.

To increase workload, add ankle and/or wristweights.

THE EXERCISE CYCLE AND ROWER PROGRAMMES

Because there are so many different makes of exercise cycle and rowing machines, all offering varying degrees of sophistication, resistance and so on, your three-stage programme should be guided by the instructions that come with your cycle/rower.

But the theory remains the same – gradually increase the workload on your machine so that you have to work harder to achieve the same distance covered in the same time – or you have to pedal faster and thus cover more distance in the same time. Work out your programme so that you spend your time on the cycle/rower feeling slightly breathless but not over-exerted and so that you can keep up a steady pace for the middle 16 minutes of your programme. The first 2 minutes and last 2 minutes should be slower – warming up and cooling down.

THE STEP/SKIP REBOUND PROGRAMME

Note: This programme is probably the best bet if you are for any reason tied to the home and if you don't own an exercise cycle or rower. It combines stepping up and down onto a stair, skipping using an ordinary rope, and rebounding (using a mini-trampoline) which is optional. Rebounders, including a hand support, are now readily available and inexpensive and are particularly useful for people with joint problems, including arthritis, who can't get to a swimming pool, as they offer low-impact aerobic exercise.

If you don't wish to buy a rebounder you can substitute stair climbing for this section of the programme – simply going up and down stairs as fast as you can for the prescribed period.

The step can be done either on a very sturdy wooden box or stool or using the bottom stair of the flight. The *step* is performed as in your *AM* PLAN warm-up described on page 162. *Skip* on alternate feet. *Rebound* by making small jumps into the air at the centre of your rebounder. Wear shorts or leggings and a T-shirt, and comfortable trainers.

Stage One

- First 2 minutes – slow jogging on spot to warm up.
- Next 2 minutes – step.
- Next 2 minutes – skip slowly.
- Next 2 minutes – rebound jumping.
- Next 2 minutes – slow jogging on spot.
- Now repeat step/skip/rebound programme for the full 20 minutes if you can, ending with a minute slow jogging on spot to cool down. If you can't manage the full programme at first, just do what you can. Remember, you should be pleasantly breathless during this routine, not gasping for breath or in any discomfort.

Stage Two
- First 2 minutes – slow skipping to warm up.
- Next 5 minutes – step.
- Next 5 minutes – rebound jumping.
- Next 5 minutes – brisk skipping.
- Next 3 minutes – step and slow jog to cool down.

Stage Three
- First 2 minutes – steady skipping to warm up.
- Next 5 minutes – very brisk step.
- Next 5 minutes – high rebound jumping.
- Next 5 minutes – brisk skipping.
- Next 2 minutes – brisk step then 1-minute steady skip to cool down.

Once you can complete Stage Three well, wear ankle and wristweights to increase the workload.

Additional activities

As well as your 20-minute *PM* PLAN six days a week, you may also consider adding other sports or pastimes to your life to increase your activity levels even more. Sports such as golf, tennis and badminton are not really aerobic sports as they don't involve raising the heart rate for long enough periods of time – however they will burn up calories and help to tone you up, so anything extra that you enjoy is well worth doing.

For fun, check out the list here to see how many

calories per minute extra (on *top* of your resting metabolic rate which is approximately 1 calorie a minute on average) you will burn up by doing a variety of activities.

CALORIE BURN-UP CHART

Activity	Extra calories burnt per minute*
Aerobics class	6
Badminton	4
Cycling, brisk	8
Dancing, disco	4
Digging garden	5
Golf	4
Gymnastics	4
Hiking with back-pack, steady	4
Horse riding, trot	4
Horse riding, walk	2
Housework, heavy	3
Jogging, 8 mph	3
Mowing grass	3
Netball, average game	6
Roller skating, fast	5
Rowing, steady	6
Rugby and football, active	7
Skiing, downhill	7
Skipping, fast	8
Squash, fast	12

Stair climbing, walking	6
running	10
Swimming, fast crawl	8
breast-stroke	7
Table tennis, moderate	4
Tennis, moderate	6
Walking, slow	2
Walking, medium	4
Walking, brisk	5
Weightlifting	8
Yoga	2

*For a person weighing 10 stone. If you weigh more you will use more, if you weigh less you will use less.

CHAPTER SEVEN

Now Be Slim for Life

There is no doubt about it – keeping slim is, for most people, even harder than getting slim. So the first piece of good news I am going to give you, the newly slim person, is that because you have dieted down to target weight on the *High Speed Slimming* system, you are not going to find staying slim a problem this time *if* you read this chapter and obey some very simple guidelines. The second piece of good news is that there is no truth in the often-cited idea that weight lost quickly has more chance of returning than weight lost slowly. And the third piece of good news is that you will *not* have to exist on a measly 1000 calories or so a day to maintain your new weight. Even without the metabolism-speeding practices that you've learnt in *High Speed Slimming* – which I hope you will continue now that you *are* slim – research shows that 'post-obese' people (i.e. people who were once fat and now are not) do *not* have slower metabolisms than people of the same weight who have never been fat.

A scientific study conducted by the Dunn Clinical Nutrition Centre in Cambridge and published in 1990 in the Proceedings of the Nutrition Society proved this. They studied a group of post-obese women who had lost an average of over 4 stone each and compared them with a second group of women similar in age and height who had never been over-weight and a third group of women who were still overweight. They discovered that the post-obese women had an average of just over 1 400 calories a day resting metabolic rate and a total daily energy expenditure of 2 230 – both figures slightly higher than those for the always-lean group!

The scientists came to the conclusion that 'many post-obese claim that they have to consume a lower energy intake to maintain the same weight as those who have never been obese. These results do not support the contention …'

So why then do so many people claim that they have to eat like a bird to stay slim? There is a simple explanation. As the Dunn Clinic observed in the report mentioned above, 'the post-obese have lower absolute energy requirements *compared with their obese state* because of the change in their weight.' Going back to their comparison trials, the still-obese women of the same age and height as the no-longer-obese and always-lean groups used up many more calories a day *just because they were fat*. Their RMRs averaged 1 603 calories a day – over 200 more than the post-obese women, and their total daily energy expenditure averaged 2 461.

In other words, when you are slim, all other

things being equal, you will need hundreds fewer calories than you did when you were fat. *Slim people eat less than fat people*. But once-fat people *don't* have to eat less than always-slim people.

The truth is that newly slim people often convince themselves that they are eating next to nothing because they are eating less than they used to when fat. But, those Dunn studied above show quite clearly that a woman who has lost four stone and now weighs 10 stone can eat well over 2000 calories a day and maintain her new weight.

If your target weight happened to be much lower than this – say, you are now 8 stone – your total daily energy expenditure is likely to be 200 or so less than this figure, but you are still going to be able to eat much more than a dieting level of calories and stay slim.

So the first thing to do when thinking about weight maintenance is to stop kidding yourself that you won't be able to eat a thing – you can and will.

KEYS TO WEIGHT MAINTENANCE

I consider the four key areas to successful weight maintenance to be *a metabolism-boosting lifestyle; knowledge of how your body behaves and of what makes a healthy diet; common sense* and *motivation*. Let's take these four key areas one by one.

Metabolism-boosting lifestyle

As explained above, *all things being equal*, the slim person will be eating fewer calories a day than she or he did when fat in order to maintain her/his new figure.

However, as I showed in Chapter Three, if the slim person makes an effort to increase her/his metabolic rate by a variety of simple means, she or he could actually end up with a metabolic rate FASTER than it was when she/he was fat!

So the single most sensible thing you, the newly-slim person, can do to maintain your new size is to continue practising all those metabolism-boosters that helped you to slim so easily. It is the diet, exercise and lifestyle philosophies described in detail in Chapter Three that will do MOST to help you maintain your new weight for life. They should be second nature to you by now after losing weight with *High Speed Slimming*. If not, go back and read them again.

Here are the main points to remember:

DIET:

• Eat plenty of 'complex carbohydrates' – grains, pulses, root vegetables, seeds, fresh fruit and vegetables. Always aim to get around 60% of your daily calories in the form of these foods. Aim to get from 15–20% of calories as protein and from 20–25% of calories as fat. (On a maintenance diet you needn't keep your fat intake quite as low as 20% if you don't want to.)

- Eat frequently and don't go more than 2½ hours without food. The snacking/high carbohydrate principle will banish food cravings and hunger pangs from your life for good.

- Eat more earlier in the day and avoid huge meals late in the evening.

- Eat plenty of raw foods, vitamin C-rich foods and spicy foods.

LIFESTYLE:

- Be a fidgeter – be more active in your daily life.

- Don't sleep longer than necessary.

- Get plenty of fresh air into your lungs and keep cool.

- Enjoy life.

EXERCISE:

Maintaining a regular exercise routine will do more than almost anything else to ensure you stay slim for the rest of your life. It burns off many calories while you do it; it speeds up your metabolism for a long time afterwards; and it builds lean tissue which burns more calories than fat tissue.

So please, *do* continue with the *AM* PLAN and the *PM* PLAN. Doing them six days a week as you did while slimming will ensure that you can eat hundreds of calories more a day than if you did nothing. Doing them even three times a week will make a considerable contribution. You could alter-nate the *AM* PLAN with the *PM* PLAN – doing one one day, the other the next.

Twenty minutes a day isn't hard to find if you want to find it. (If you are in doubt about that – read the section on motivation!)

Knowledge

What many diets don't tell you is that once you begin eating more again, you will experience an almost inevitable gain in weight of around 3 lbs. This is the body restoring its levels of fluid and glycogen – just as it lost them first when you began the diet. This weight gain is *not* fat. But as many dieters don't know this, they see a few pounds weight gain on the scales the minute, so it appears, that they've finished the diet – and they assume that it is fat, and that they will continue to put on pounds of weight every week and soon be back where they began '... so I might as well give up and start bingeing again'.

The glycogen gain is a one-off gain, so don't give up in despair because of it. Next week there won't be a gain, nor any other week after that if you just eat normally. My favourite way of coping with the glycogen gain in the first week after coming off a diet is to end the diet a couple of pounds lower than you would ideally like to be – so that once the glycogen levels are restored you are *then* what you want to be.

What many diets also don't tell you is how or

what to eat when the slimming is finished. So you are left floundering and it is no wonder that many people fail to maintain the loss.

After *High Speed Slimming*, *what* you eat is easy – you simply carry on eating the same type of diet – high in complex carbohydrates, reasonably high in protein and low in fat. Luckily, the *High Speed Slimming* way of eating not only helps boost metabolism, but it is also a healthy, palatable, varied way to eat long-term. There's nothing more boring than counting calories every day for the rest of your life and there is absolutely no need to. You could, if you like, follow Plan One, but increase portion sizes to suit yourself. Or you can just follow these diet guidelines then use the 'traffic light' food listings below to maintain your weight loss.

• Build up to eating more gradually. For instance, if you finished *High Speed Slimming* on Plan Three or Four, you could spend a week eating on Plan One or Two, then the following week you could add a few hundred calories a day or so of extra foods – preferably extra carbohydrates such as bread, potatoes, rice or pasta.

• The simple way to tell if you are eating properly is to weigh yourself once a week. If you have put on any weight then you are beginning to eat a little too much; if you have lost weight, you are not eating quite enough. The only exception to this is that most women will gain a few pounds in the few days before their period — this gain is fluid, will disappear in a week or so, and should be discounted.

• Try to eat a diet as high in natural unprocessed foods as you can. Processing often hides fat, sugar and calories and removes the fibre from food. If you eat many packaged convenience foods, read the labels and try to avoid the ones which list fats or oils high up in the list of ingredients. Go for products labelled 'high in fibre' and 'low in fat'. And if there is a nutrition panel on the pack, which should list carbohydrate, fat and protein content per 100g of product, see if the balance is anywhere near the 60-20-20 of the *High Speed Slimming* system. Plenty of fresh fruits, salads and vegetables will fill you up without adding too many calories. But now you are maintaining weight, you can alter the balance slightly to 60-15-25 if you like — eating a little less protein by percentage and a little more fat. (Though of course as you are now eating many more calories a day than you did when slimming, you will actually be eating *more* protein so there is never any problem.) For example, 20% of the calories in a 1000 calories a day diet equals 50g of protein — 15% of the calories in a 2,000 calories a day diet equals 75g of protein. Keep thinking 'more carbohydrates' and 'less fat' and you need never count calories again.

• Remember tasty meals need not be high in calories — use plenty of herbs and spices in your maintenance diet.

Now follow the *Traffic Light Plan* as an easy, no-fuss way to eat all you like without putting on weight.

The Traffic Light Maintenance Diet

GREEN: The foods listed below should form the bulk of your daily diet because they are low, or reasonably low, in calories, high in nutrients and will maintain your diet in 60-20-20 balance easily.

Fresh fruit
All fresh salad items
All fresh vegetables – raw or cooked without fat
Potatoes
Wholegrain breads
Wholewheat pasta
Brown rice
Lentils, kidney beans and other pulses
Baked beans
Bulgar (cracked wheat)
Wholegrain breakfast cereals without added sugar
Natural low-fat yogurt
White fish
Prawns
Crab
Chicken
Turkey
Game
Liver
Cottage cheese
Skimmed milk soft cheese
Vegeburgers

Fromage frais
Skimmed milk
Eggs
Very lean red meat

AMBER: The remainder of your diet should be made up mostly from this list. They too contain nutrients but tend to be higher in calories so it is worth eating them with 'caution'.

Wholemeal pastry items
Fresh nuts
Crispbreads
Medium fat cheeses
Wholemilk and fruit yogurts
Oily fish, fresh or canned
Dried fruits
Avocado
Low-fat spread
Fruit juices
Canned fruits
Fruit spreads
Vegetable pâté
Tinned soups

RED: Think of the following foods as the ones to use sparingly or eat occasionally on your diet. Most are high in fat and/or low on nutrients and eating too many of them will upset your diet's 60-20-20 balance.

Eat sparingly:
Butter
Margarine
Cooking oils
Salad oils
Oily dressings
Peanut butter
Tinned meats
Deli meats
Bacon and gammon
Sausages
Cream
High-fat cheese, e.g. full-fat cream cheese, Stilton
Ice cream and chilled desserts
Sugared cereals
Crisps
Salted nuts
Chips

Eat VERY sparingly:
Chocolates
Sweets
Gateaux
Puddings
Biscuits
Battered, deep-fried foods
Pastries, Pasties and Pies

Common sense

It is amazing how many otherwise-sensible people who run big businesses, raise several children perfectly or are world champions in their field, go to pieces at the thought of organizing their own diets. Yet eating well, slimly and healthily, is largely a matter of common sense. From day to day, if you choose a wide variety of foods from the *Green* and *Amber* lists above, you'll be getting a good diet. If one day you know (and everybody *does* know!) that you've eaten more than you should, all you do is cut down a little bit the next day.

And what of the people for whom a routine is the exception? If you entertain a lot or travel a lot, so I am often told, you can't watch what you eat. Well, I believe you can if you want to. Most of the problem is that people don't think ahead. If you're on the road a lot, for instance, the best food of all is food you have had the foresight to buy and prepare yourself at home. With the right containers, flasks, etc., you can take virtually any food with you – not just sandwiches, but a variety of salads and soups. For ideas, go back to the menus in Chapter 4 and the recipes in Chapter Five.

If you have to entertain frequently in restaurants, always make your restaurant meal your main meal of the day, try to pick a restaurant you know, where you can get food that isn't high in fat, and use common sense about avoiding the *Red* foods. When I go out for a meal for pleasure, I always eat what I like because it doesn't happen that often. However, because I am now so used to eating in the 60-20-20 way, I usually find that without even thinking about it, I have chosen a meal that more or less fits in with that ideal.

If you enjoy wine or other alcohol, you can have that, too. I would say a sensible limit is *two* bottles of wine a week – that's equivalent to 10 glasses – or 10 large measures of spirit or 5 pints of beer, lager or cider a week.

Oh dear – weight gain!

And what do you do if the unthinkable happens – you have put on a few pounds? The first thing to do is not panic. The second thing to do is not to ignore it. Do something about it – now. Either cut back generally for a few days or, if you need something more structured, go back on to whichever plan you began dieting on in *High Speed Slimming* until you have lost those few pounds again.

Ask yourself *why* you put on those few pounds. It could be that you lack …

Motivation

Let me return to Professor Arnold Bender, the world-famous obesity specialist who is now a consultant to the Weight Watchers organization. Remember, earlier in this book his comments confirmed my suspicions that there is no physical or scientific reason why people who lose weight quickly should put it back on quickly, or be more inclined than anyone else to put weight back on at all.

I'd now like to tell you what else he said.

'People who manage to maintain their weight successfully are the people who keep themselves highly motivated. For example, of *nine thousand* Weight Watchers lecturers in the USA, *nine thousand* have kept their weight off. Their motivation is strong – they lose their jobs if they *don't* keep it off.

'Incentive and motivation are what is needed. Most people can supply that incentive by looking back at all the reasons they wanted to lose weight in the first place, and saying, "Well, if I put weight back on, look at what I'll lose".'

Losing weight can be like studying for an Open University degree – getting there is fun. But once there – what next? Just as many people put their degree certificate in a drawer and forget it, so many slimmers lose motivation because they don't do anything with their new selves. So the moment you are slim – or whenever you feel the 'why bother?' syndrome coming on – write yourself a list of all the good things that being slim does for you. Here are some suggestions that might spark off your own ideas:

- Being slim gives me added confidence — it helps me talk to people and make new friends.
- Being slim gives other people a different view of me.
- Being slim has made me take an interest in clothes and in being smart for the first time in years.
- Being slim makes me feel fitter and healthier.
- Being slim makes me feel, 'If I've done this, I can do almost anything!'
- Being slim has improved my sex life.

And so on! So if you put on weight again, presumably all these marvellous benefits (or your own version of them) will disappear.

Surely the key to life-long slimness, then, is to *build* on the benefits that being slim has given you. Let's see what you can do.

Being slim has given you more confidence. So now look at what you might be able to do that you didn't feel you could do before. Apply for a better job? Sign up for an evening class in something you always wanted to learn? Start up a local group of your own?

You feel fitter and healthier. Right — so now how about taking up an exciting sport — scuba diving or orienteering? Something you couldn't do before, but now you could. How about joining a health club, or taking a teaching course in exercise to music?

The point is — slimness is just the start of endless possibilities. In my experience, many (though of course, not all) overweight people ignore the possibilities life holds – somehow being fat and being a 'viewer', not a 'doer', go together.

I'm not saying life is going to be perfect from now on – of course it isn't. But your new-found confidence can be used, again, to *take* disappointments, unfairness and setbacks and get over them *without* using the fat person's mental attitude of 'What's the use of trying – things always go wrong ...' and then turning to food as a silent friend. Food as comfort, believe me, is the silent *enemy*. Use food – don't let it use you.

You – yes, *you* – can be slim for life, starting today!

Sphere now offers an exciting range of quality titles by both established and new authors. All of the books in this series are available from:

Sphere Books,
Cash Sales Department,
P.O. Box 11,
Falmouth,
Cornwall TR10 9EN.

Alternatively you may fax your order to the above address. Fax No. 0326 376423.

Payments can be made as follows: Cheque, postal order (payable to Macdonald & Co (Publishers) Ltd) or by credit cards, Visa/Access. Do not send cash or currency. UK customers and B.F.P.O.: please send a cheque or postal order (no currency) and allow £1.00 for postage and packing for the first book, plus 50p for the second book, plus 30p for each additional book up to a maximum charge of £3.00 (7 books plus).

Overseas customers including Ireland, please allow £2.00 for postage and packing for the first book, plus £1.00 for the second book, plus 50p for each additional book.

NAME (Block Letters) ....

ADDRESS ....

....

☐ I enclose my remittance for _____

☐ I wish to pay by Access/Visa Card

Number ⬜⬜⬜⬜⬜.⬜⬜⬜⬜⬜⬜⬜⬜⬜⬜⬜⬜⬜

Card Expiry Date ⬜⬜⬜⬜